Men's Body Sculpting

Second Edition

Nick Evans, MD, FRCS

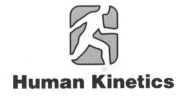

Human Kinetics

Library of Congress Cataloging-in-Publication Data

Evans, Nick, 1964-
  Men's body sculpting / Nick Evans. -- 2nd ed.
     p. cm.
  Includes bibliographical references and index.
  ISBN-13: 978-0-7360-8321-8 (softcover)
  ISBN-10: 0-7360-8321-9 (softcover)
  1. Bodybuilding. I. Title.
  GV546.5.E83 2010
  613.7'13--dc22

                                2010027748

ISBN-10: 0-7360-8321-9 (print)
ISBN-13: 978-0-7360-8321-8 (print)

Acquisitions Editor: Justin Klug; **Developmental Editor:** Anne Hall; **Assistant Editors:** Elizabeth Evans, Cory Weber; **Copyeditor:** Patricia L. MacDonald; **Indexer:** Dan Connolly; **Graphic Designer:** Joe Buck; **Graphic Artist:** Francine Hamerski; **Cover Designer:** Keith Blomberg; **Photographer (cover):** iStockphoto/Damir Spanic; **Photographer (interior):** Nigel Farrow; **Visual Production Assistant:** Joyce Brumfield; **Photo Production Manager:** Jason Allen; **Art Manager:** Kelly Hendren; **Associate Art Manager:** Alan L. Wilborn; **Illustrator:** Jason M. McAlexander, MFA; **Printer:** United Graphics

Human Kinetics books are available at special discounts for bulk purchase. Special editions or book excerpts can also be created to specification. For details, contact the Special Sales Manager at Human Kinetics.

Printed in the United States of America   10 9 8 7 6 5 4 3 2 1

The paper in this book is certified under a sustainable forestry program.

Human Kinetics

Web site: www.HumanKinetics.com

United States: Human Kinetics
P.O. Box 5076
Champaign, IL 61825-5076
800-747-4457
e-mail: humank@hkusa.com

Canada: Human Kinetics
475 Devonshire Road Unit 100
Windsor, ON N8Y 2L5
800-465-7301 (in Canada only)
e-mail: info@hkcanada.com

Europe: Human Kinetics
107 Bradford Road
Stanningley
Leeds LS28 6AT, United Kingdom
+44 (0) 113 255 5665
e-mail: hk@hkeurope.com

Australia: Human Kinetics
57A Price Avenue
Lower Mitcham, South Australia 5062
08 8372 0999
e-mail: info@hkaustralia.com

New Zealand: Human Kinetics
P.O. Box 80
Torrens Park, South Australia 5062
0800 222 062
e-mail: info@hknewzealand.com

E4811

Men's Body Sculpting

Second Edition

Contents

Exercise Finder. vi

Preface ix

Acknowledgments xi

PART I   BODY-SCULPTING SCIENCE **1**

    Chapter 1   Rules to Lift By 3

    Chapter 2   Feeding the Machine 13

    Chapter 3   Meet the Muscles 27

    Chapter 4   Program Prescription. 37

PART II   MAXIMIZING MUSCLE MASS **43**

    Chapter 5   Mass Construction. 45

    Chapter 6   Gaining an Anabolic Advantage. 53

    Chapter 7   Mass Generator Program 61

PART III   CUTTING BODY FAT **81**

    Chapter 8   Lean Muscle Training 83

    Chapter 9   Gaining a Lean Advantage. 91

    Chapter 10 Body Fat Blitz Program 99

PART IV CHISELING THE ULTIMATE BODY **121**

Chapter 11 Climbing the Ladder of Intensity 123

Chapter 12 Anabolic Overdrive 133

Chapter 13 Supplement Stack 143

Chapter 14 Hybrid Hard Body Program 151

PART V MUSCLE MAINTENANCE **189**

Chapter 15 Advanced Sculpting Solutions and Training Tips . . .191

Chapter 16 Sculpting Safely 201

Chapter 17 Survival Strategies for the Peak Physique 215

Appendix A   Training, Progress, and Nutrition Charts 229

Appendix B   Food Nutrition Facts 233

Bibliography 234

Index 237

About the Author 243

Exercise Finder

Exercise	Equipment used	Chapter	Page
Chest			
Dumbbell chest fly	2 dumbbells	7	67
Incline bench press	Barbell	7	68
Cable crossover	Cable crossover machine	10	105
Incline dumbbell press	2 dumbbells; incline bench	10	106
Machine chest fly	Chest fly machine	14	157
Machine incline press	Smith machine	14	158
Decline bench press	2 dumbbells; decline bench	14	159
Shoulders			
Dumbbell lateral raise	2 dumbbells	7	69
Barbell shoulder press	Barbell	7	70
Seated dumbbell lateral raise	2 dumbbells; exercise bench	10	107
Dumbbell shoulder press	2 dumbbells; exercise bench	10	108
Machine upright row	Deltoid raise machine	14	181
Rear deltoid fly	Deltoid fly machine	14	182
Front deltoid raise	Dumbbell	14	183
Back			
Chin-up	Overhead bar	7	77
Barbell row	Barbell	7	78
Wide-grip pull-down	Cable pull-down machine	10	109
Seated cable row	Seated row machine	10	110
Reverse-grip pull-down	Cable pull-down machine	14	164
Dumbbell row	Dumbbell; exercise bench	14	165
Lumbar extension	Extension bench	14	166
Biceps			
Barbell curl	Barbell	7	79
Dumbbell curl	2 dumbbells	10	111
Preacher curl	Dumbbell; preacher bench	14	167
Concentration curl	Dumbbell; exercise bench	14	168
Triceps			
Close-grip bench press	Barbell	7	71
Triceps push-down	Cable machine	10	112
Triceps dip	Parallel bars	14	160
One-arm triceps push-down	High pulley machine	14	161

Exercise	Equipment used	Chapter	Page
Quadriceps			
Leg extension	Leg extension machine	7, 14	73,171
Barbell squat	Barbell; squat rack	7	74
Unilateral leg extension	Leg extension machine	10	115
Machine squat	Smith machine	10	116
Leg press	Leg press machine	14	172
Machine squat	Squat machine	14	173
Hamstrings			
Leg curl	Leg curl machine	7	75
Unilateral leg curl	Upright leg curl machine	10	117
Leg curl	Leg curl machine	14	174
Straight-leg deadlift	Barbell	14	175
Calves			
Standing calf raise	Standing calf raise machine	7	76
Donkey calf raise	Calf block; exercise bench	10	118
Seated calf raise	Seated calf machine	14	176
Straight-leg calf raise	Leg press machine	14	177
Abs			
Decline sit-up	Decline bench	7	72
Incline leg raise	Abdominal bench	7	80
Twisting sit-up	Decline bench	10	113
Vertical leg raise	Vertical leg raise apparatus	10	114
Floor crunch	Floor mat (optional)	10	119
Dumbbell pullover	Dumbbell; exercise bench	10	120
Rope crunch	High pulley machine	14	162
Cable side crunch	High pulley cable machine	14	163
Machine crunch	Abdominal crunch machine	14	185
Bench leg raise	Exercise bench	14	186
Forearms			
Barbell wrist curl	Barbell; exercise bench	14	169
Reverse wrist curl	Barbell; exercise bench	14	170
Rotator cuff			
External rotation	Cable pulley machine	14	178
Internal rotation	Cable pulley machine	14	179
Cable lateral raise	Cable pulley machine	14	180
Trapezius			
Shrug	2 dumbbells	14	184

Preface

Picture the perfect body, the kind of body you really want. Now hold that thought. What do you see? A sleek six-pack? Awesome arms? Bold shoulders and a chiseled chest? An image of physical perfection? Well, that dream body *could* be yours. The secret is right here in this book.

All you must do is make a simple decision, right here, right now. You have two choices: One, put the book down and walk away empty-handed, or two, take the book home and absorb the power within its pages.

It's a no-brainer, really, but think for a minute anyway. It's no coincidence that this book caught your eye, that you picked it from the shelf, that you're holding it in your hands, and that I have your attention. It's your destiny. It's your right to have the body you want, and now you have the opportunity, the chance to change, to turn your dream body into reality, to become a sculpture of living flesh and blood with bulging muscles shredding your clothes from the inside.

You'd like that, wouldn't you? Imagine a tight torso bringing a smile to your face every time you look in the mirror. Think about turning heads as you walk down the street. Think of it. What have you got to lose? Nothing ventured, nothing gained, right? Unlock the door to your true potential. Make a difference before it's too late.

Okay, time's up. You decide. What's it going to be? Read the book and say hello to your new custom-built body or . . . well, there isn't really another option, is there? You know it's time to get the body you want. It's a decision you'll never regret. Within these pages you'll find everything you want to know about building a stronger, leaner, more muscular physique.

As of yet, there's no magic pill for developing a body of armor. (If you know of one, can you pick me up a lifetime supply?) You can't gulp down the latest nutritional supplement and expect an instant transformation. You can't just walk into a department store on Memorial Day and buy a fashionable physique for the summer. There's more to gaining muscle than walking through the doors of a gym, listening to the clang of iron, the whir of stationary bikes, and the grunts of other people bench pressing.

I know you probably know your way around a gym. But if you're tired of spending countless hours pumping iron with little or no change in your physique, this book will save you time, effort, and money by revealing the most direct route to your physical perfection. End your frustration and start achieving results in a fraction of the time. Make no mistake—this isn't a pop-up picture book of exercises or a quick-fix boot camp for couch potatoes. This is the real deal; basic training is over and we're on the battlefield. So, lock and load your muscles. Take aim at your body fat, and get ready for a massive attack. Your mission—if you choose to accept it—is staged in five integrated steps: Part I includes the basic scientific principles that underpin any successful body sculpting program; part II explains the methods you can use to maximize muscle mass; part III teaches how to cut body fat for a lean physique; part IV details the steps you'll need to hone your muscles into a chiseled form using diet and exercise; and part V is a guide to maintaining the figure you've worked so hard to achieve for lasting results.

If you're one of the millions of people worldwide who work out, this is a book you can't afford to be without. It's a must for your gym bag. Everything you need to know in order to tweak your technique and fine-tune your physique is in these pages. Life is not a dress rehearsal. There's no rewind button. You get only one body, one chance, and the clock is ticking. What are you waiting for?

Acknowledgments

I wish to thank the following individuals and organizations for their help on this book:

Human Kinetics for creative and technical guidance

Nigel Farrow for his enthusiastic photography

Models James, Tim, and Terry for helping demonstrate the exercises

Compass Gym, Scarborough, England for providing the photo-shoot location

And thanks to all the readers who purchased the first edition of this book.

Body-Sculpting Science

In part I, you'll learn the basic scientific principles that hold the key to successful body sculpting. Part I is the gateway to the book—all readers are advised to study this section before proceeding. Right away (chapter 1) you'll learn the best exercise techniques to stimulate muscle growth. The next time you set foot in the gym, you'll have a new set of rules to lift by, with brutal assault tactics to raise the intensity level of your workouts. Armed with these trade secrets, you'll have no excuse for not reaching your potential. Exercise requires high-grade muscle fuel. For the bodybuilder, the challenge is to provide the right nutrients to feed muscle growth while starving the fat stores at the same time. In chapter 2, you'll find winning recipes for a hard muscle diet and my secret ingredients for getting that shredded six-pack. In chapter 3, you'll learn everything you need to know about anatomy so you'll be able to customize your body with surgical precision. In chapter 4, you'll find out how to choose the correct body-sculpting program for your own individual body type.

Rules to Lift By

It seems like a simple concept—lift weights to make your muscles grow bigger and stronger—but there's so much more to it than meets the eye. In fact, one could say, "You think you know about muscle growth? You have no idea!"

For instance, when it comes to maximizing muscle growth, do you know how many repetitions you should perform or how much weight you should lift? Should you lift the weight slowly or quickly? What is the optimal number of sets? How long should you rest between sets? How long does it take for your muscles to recover between workouts? What's happening inside your muscles when they grow? What exactly does *intensity* mean? What is momentary muscular failure?

You might know your way around a weight room, and you've probably spent countless hours working out, but have you ever stopped to think about precisely what you're doing and why you're doing it that way? It's easy to switch on autopilot and cruise through your workout, but is your routine really working for you? Are you seeing changes in your physique? Or, are you frustrated by your lack of progress?

Instead of going nowhere with the same old business-as-usual training routine, maybe it's time to pause and gather your thoughts. Take a class on muscle mass. After all, if you know why muscles grow, you'll understand how to make it happen. Remember that your body is a masterpiece of biology—learn to work with nature, not against it.

I'll show you what works and what doesn't so that you won't get stuck in first gear at the gym. Using my five-point checklist, you'll be able to systematically evaluate your workouts and tune up your training technique like a master mechanic. The next time you hit the gym, you'll drive through the doors with a new set of rules to lift by and surefire tactics for monster mass.

What Money Can't Buy

Are you familiar with the credit card commercials on TV that list a bunch of purchases and their values? In your case, the ad would probably go something like this:

Gym membership—$395; lifting belt—$39; tight tank top—$25; latest nutritional supplement—$46; shredding your shirtsleeves with bulging biceps—priceless!

MUSCLE GROWTH

Muscle growth requires three things: stimulus, fuel, and repair. The stimulus—exercise—makes the muscle work, drains its energy store, and causes microscopic damage to the muscle fibers. After exercise, the muscle must replenish its fuel tank and repair itself. Provided that the stimulus was of sufficient intensity, the muscle will adapt (grow) during the repair process.

Muscle adapts to exercise so that it is better equipped and functionally more effective when it receives the next bout of exercise. The three types of adaptation are neural, hypertrophic, and metabolic. An increase in muscle strength is largely due to neural adaptation, which enhances the muscle's electrical supply. The nerve impulses fire more quickly and recruit more muscle fibers, resulting in a more powerful muscular contraction. Initial strength gains from weight training reflect neural adaptations, but, in the long term, improvements in strength are secondary to an increase in muscle size. In other words, strength follows size.

An increase in muscle size is due to hypertrophic adaptation, which results in an increase in the cross-sectional area of individual muscle fibers. Exercise-induced hypertrophy affects fast-twitch Type II (strength) fibers more than it affects slow-twitch Type I (endurance) fibers. So as the muscle gets bigger, it becomes stronger.

During metabolic adaptation, the muscle's biochemical profile evolves to improve oxygen and energy use. This process improves muscular endurance.

The strength–endurance continuum is a theory that explains how muscle undergoes a specific adaptation to an imposed demand. At one end, strength training induces primarily neural adaptations; at the opposite end, endurance training causes metabolic changes. Hypertrophic adaptations are induced by training methods that exist somewhere between the two extremes—hence, the concept of task specificity. If you want pure muscle strength, train like a weightlifter. If you prefer muscular endurance, train like a long-distance runner. If your primary goal is size, your muscle requires a different set of imposed demands. You don't want your muscle to adapt via purely neural pathways or metabolic pathways. What you need is hypertrophic adaptation, which creates bigger muscles, more mass, and monster size.

To generate a hypertrophic response, the exercise stimulus must be intense. Exercise intensity is the degree of effort, or the percentage of momentary ability. At the point of momentary muscular failure, an effort of 100 percent intensity is required to complete the last rep. The muscle is pushed to its functional limit and must contract to its maximum capability to complete the task. Performing a set to failure generates 100 percent intensity, and the magnitude of this huge stimulus results in hypertrophic adaptation. If you want muscular growth, you must work the muscle to the point of failure.

During exercise, muscle gets its energy from a substance called adenosine triphosphate (ATP). This unit of energy has three sources—phosphocreatine, glycogen, and oxygen—that act in sequence, like a trail of dominos. When you begin your first repetition, phosphocreatine provides the energy. This stuff is stored inside muscle, ready for action, but its supply lasts only up to 10 seconds. After that point, glycogen takes over as the energy provider. The chemical conversion of glycogen releases lactic acid as a by-product, and it's this buildup of acid in the muscle that inflicts a burning pain and leads to fatigue within two to three minutes.

These first two energy sources are anaerobic—that is, they do not require oxygen. At the completion of one set to failure, your fatigued muscles scream with the pain of excess acid. Your breathing gets heavy as you gasp for the third source of energy—oxygen. Blood flow into the muscle increases, delivering the much-needed oxygen to relieve the oxygen debt and wash out the lactic acid buildup. This rush of blood inflates the muscle like a balloon, causing the phenomenon known as the muscle pump.

An intense set of repetitions performed to the point of muscular failure is an insult to the muscle. This not only depletes the muscle's energy store but also causes microscopic damage to the muscle tissue. These disrupted muscle fibers cause delayed-onset muscle soreness, the muscular pain that peaks a day or two after intense exercise. During the recovery phase, the muscle's energy stores of glycogen and phosphocreatine are restocked from dietary carbohydrate and creatine. The damaged muscle fibers are repaired by protein synthesis using dietary amino acids. The repair process regenerates a bigger muscle fiber.

Fiber disruption is essential for muscular hypertrophy. It takes five to seven days to repair the muscle damage induced by high-intensity weight training. After an all-out assault on your muscles, an adequate period of rest is essential if you want to build those muscle fibers.

The general adaptation syndrome theory suggests that a body system will adapt with improved function when faced with a stress to which it is not accustomed. This concept implies that when the neuromuscular system is overloaded, it adapts to match the stress, but if the stress is left unchanged over time, adaptation will reach a plateau. The principle of overload is of paramount importance if you want to continue growing muscle. That's why lifting weights is properly termed progressive resistance training. Once your muscle adapts to lifting a certain weight, you make it work harder by progressing to the next level of stimulus by increasing the resistance. If you do not elicit an overload effect, hypertrophic adaptation will cease. Adaptation to a training stimulus deteriorates within two weeks of exposure. To maximize neuromuscular adaptation, the stimulus—such as load—should be increased every two to three weeks.

Now that you know why muscles grow, your next step is to put the principles you have learned into practice. Let's turn our discussion to what you have to do at the gym to generate the precise stimulus that induces hypertrophic adaptation in your muscles.

LIFTING GUIDELINES

For even the simplest task there are usually several ways to get the job done. Let's say I give you three objects: a hammer, a nail, and a piece of wood. How will you go about hitting the nail into the wood? Maybe you'll take the cautious approach and hit the nail repetitively with many gentle taps of the hammer, sinking the nail into the wood slowly but surely, taking a few moments to complete the task. Alternatively, you could strike the nail a single time with all your might, sinking it into the wood with one huge blow, completing the task in one second. The second approach is far quicker in terms of time and effort, but there's an element of risk involved. If you miss the nail, you might bring the hammer crashing down onto your thumb with a painful thump. And that would be the end of hammering for a while.

Like driving a nail into wood, training with weights has several possible techniques. Too little weight and the exercise is ineffective—you'd get more of a workout washing your car. Too much weight and you could wind up in the emergency room with a torn muscle. What we need is middle ground. Let's sift through the bodybuilder's toolbox and select the best tools to construct your body effectively and safely.

Before you start work on your body, we'll first analyze the principles of weight training. Why? Because manipulating the principles is the key to fine-tuning your physique. Minor details make all the difference, and the secrets lie within the fine print. Tweaking your technique involves making adjustments to every aspect of your exercise program, including your number of repetitions, amount of weight, number of sets, combination of exercises, rest intervals, and workout time.

If you want to make progress, pay close attention to detail. Imagine building your dream house. You start with simple raw materials and, brick by brick, construct your perfect palace with a solid foundation from the ground up. This is how we'll create the framework of your exercise program. Each stage is critical within the architecture of the final construct; I'll explain why as we go along.

To create a mass-building regimen that works, follow these five points: precision repetition, work set, rest interval, workout time, and recovery. Each point focuses your attention on the essential details required to stimulate the maximum hypertrophic adaptation from your muscles.

Precision Repetition

The repetition, or rep, is the building block of any workout. Two aspects of the repetition need careful consideration: quality and quantity.

The quality of a repetition is determined by its execution, or the time taken to lift and lower the weight. The speed at which the rep is performed is called the repetition cadence or tempo.

Each repetition has three phases: lower, pause, and lift. The gold-standard repetition cadence uses a two-second lowering phase, a one-second pause, and a two-second lift phase. This 2-1-2 repetition cadence requires five seconds to complete the full range of motion. A very quick repetition cadence, such as a 1-1 (no pause phase), typically allows the use of a heavier weight because of the rapid acceleration during the movement. However, quick-cadence reps actually decrease intensity because excessive momentum is introduced. A rapid movement may allow for the demonstration of strength by literally throwing the weight, but this is not the optimal way to build muscle mass.

Stimulating muscle growth requires repetitions performed in a slow, precise cadence. The movement you want can be compared to the action of a spring. On the way down, the spring is being compressed. Upon reaching the bottom, the spring releases its force in a smooth upward motion. The precision repetition is controlled and smooth, never bounced, jerked, or done with momentum. This ensures that the muscle is in a state of contraction at all times. In other words, the muscle must be kept under tension throughout the movement. It's the time under tension that provides the stimulus for muscle growth. During each rep, be sure to focus your mind on the muscle contracting and nothing else.

The phases of the precision rep evolve from scientific principles. There are three types of muscle contraction: concentric, isometric, and eccentric. To gain the maximum benefit from each repetition, your muscle should experience all three types of contraction. As an example, consider this simple task. When you raise a cup from a table to your mouth, your biceps is performing a concentric, or positive, contraction. When you lower the cup back to the table, your biceps is performing an eccentric, or negative, contraction. If you hold the cup still as you walk across the kitchen, your biceps is performing an isometric, or static, contraction. Why are these distinctions important? Because your biceps muscle must work during all three phases or else you will drop the cup.

The positive (concentric) contraction is actually the weakest of the three types. Your muscle can lower more weight than it can hold still. Your muscle can hold more weight than it can lift. Thus, an eccentric contraction is stronger than an isometric contraction, which in turn is stronger than a concentric contraction. Note what happens as you perform a biceps curl. When your biceps fails during the concentric phase, and you can't lift the weight any farther, you can still hold the weight at that point. Then, when the isometric contraction fatigues, and you can't hold the weight any longer, you are still able to lower the weight under control because the eccentric contraction is stronger.

This is the science behind a precision rep. Performing the repetition in a slow, controlled manner means you do not waste muscular contraction. You make the best use of the negative, static, and positive portions of the rep. Furthermore, slowing down repetition cadence is a method of increasing intensity.

Along with the quality of the repetition, you consider the quantity of the repetition, which involves two factors: how many reps to perform and how much weight to use.

Within the muscle, muscle fibers contract under the all-or-nothing principle. In other words, fibers either contract or they don't. Contraction is not a matter of degree. It's like striking a match—either the flame ignites or it doesn't. To move any given object, your muscle contracts just enough of its fibers to get the job done. For example, your biceps must contract only a few fibers to raise an 8-ounce (240 ml) beverage, but it must bring more fibers into action to lift a 30-pound (13.5 kg) weight. To lift the heaviest possible weight, your muscle must contract all of its fibers. When this happens, the muscle receives its maximum stimulus. Maximum stimulus leads to maximum adaptation.

As discussed previously, a muscle's response to stimulation involves neural (strength), hypertrophic (size), and metabolic (endurance) adaptation. Repetitions must be performed to the point of muscular failure to elicit the maximum response. As the number of repetitions increases, the adaptive response shifts from strength to hypertrophy and then to endurance. Performing a one-repetition maximum (1RM) induces a neural adaptation that increases muscle strength. A six- to eight-repetition maximum causes a hypertrophic response that develops muscle size. When the number of repetitions climbs into double figures, the muscle experiences more of an endurance stimulus, which fails to evoke significant adaptations in size or strength.

Scientific studies indicate that the optimal hypertrophy training protocol uses a set of six to eight repetitions performed to the point of muscular failure using the heaviest possible load. The best stimulus for inducing maximum muscular hypertrophy is to lift a weight equal to 75 to 80 percent of your 1RM repeatedly to failure, until you can no longer complete another repetition. During that last all-out effort repetition, the muscle is forced to contract all of its fibers. So at the point of momentary muscular failure, the maximum stimulus has been achieved, and your muscle will grow. Table 1.1 summarizes the load required for a range of repetitions based on the weight lifted during a 1RM.

A hypertrophic training protocol consisting of six to eight repetitions to failure requires a load equivalent to 75 to 80 percent of your 1RM. Muscles grow most effectively when the maximum stimulus—muscular failure—is achieved within this rep range. Don't try to use the heaviest possible weight. Instead, select the heaviest weight you can control with perfect form. Concentrate

Table 1.1 Required Load for Number of Repetitions

Repetitions	Load (% of 1RM)
4	85
6	80
8	75
10	70
12	65

on working one muscle unaided by momentum or the assistance of other body parts. Employ and maintain flawless form throughout the set—there's no room for compromise. Remember that it's the weight on the muscle that counts, not the weight on the bar.

So, how do you select the correct resistance for an exercise? Mathematically, the weight for a given quantity of repetitions equates to a percentage of your one-rep maximum (1RM). As outlined in table 1.1, performing a 6-rep maximum to failure requires a weight that is equivalent to around 80 percent of your 1RM, 8 reps equates to 75 percent 1RM, 10 reps requires 70 percent 1RM, and 12 reps equates to 65 percent 1RM. Whenever you begin a new exercise, it's not easy to select the correct weight right away. However, you do not need to go around the gym recording your 1RM on every exercise so you can figure out the exact weight with a pocket calculator. In fact, 1RM is "1 Risky Maneuver" that carries a high chance of injury. The most common way to select the correct weight for the last set on any given exercise is to use the initial sets as a guide.

Here's how to do it. For the first warm-up set, estimate the weight that will allow you to perform 12 to 15 reps, and give it a go. If you estimated correctly, then make an appropriate weight addition for the next set that will allow you to perform about 10 reps. By now you should be getting an idea of what weight to use for your final set in order to reach failure in 6 to 8 reps. If you selected a weight that was too heavy, and you were able to squeeze out only 4 reps, make a note to choose a slightly lighter weight next time. On the other hand, if you selected a weight that was too light, and you could easily perform 8 reps without failing, you'll need to select a slightly heavier weight next time. It may take a few trial workouts before you get the weights figured out exactly—keeping a training logbook can help. It's no big deal if you don't pick the correct weight for every exercise the first time; with experience you will get the knack of knowing the correct resistance.

Work Set

Perhaps the most controversial element of any training program is the optimal number of sets required to increase muscular hypertrophy. The debate concerns whether one set to failure is a sufficient stimulus to induce maximum hypertrophic adaptation or if multiple sets are required to elicit maximal muscular gains. According to the theory of general adaptation, muscular gains would plateau after the first set. But is this really the case?

Differences in training volume represent different degrees of stress to the neuromuscular system. Training volume is calculated as follows:

$$\text{repetitions} \times \text{sets} \times \text{percentage of 1RM}$$

When a muscle moves a weight, it performs work. In technical terms, the amount of work done depends on the size of the weight and the distance the weight is moved. You can make your muscles work harder by increasing the weight or increasing the distance moved by performing more repetitions or multiple sets.

No scientific evidence suggests that a greater training volume enhances strength or hypertrophy. There appears to be no significant difference in terms of muscular gains as a result of training with single versus multiple sets. Increases in muscle size and strength have been measured using single-set and multiple-set training; apparently, each method elicits similar neuromuscular adaptations. The question is which system represents the optimal amount of stress (volume) to induce maximal muscular adaptations? Strength increases will occur with the first set, but multiple sets may result in greater size gains. However, size and strength gains appear to follow the principle of diminished returns. With increases in training volume, the magnitude of adaptation may slow or diminish.

So can you really stimulate muscle hypertrophy with a single set to failure? In other words, can you walk into the gym, load up the bar with a weight equivalent to 80 percent of your 1RM, perform six reps to failure, and stimulate growth in every fiber of the muscle? The answer in practical terms is probably not. At the very least, you'd benefit from a warm-up set (or two) to get your muscle in the groove for that all-out maximal effort work set. In reality, you do need more than one set to recruit and exhaust all the fibers within a muscle. However, even though you perform a couple of sets to warm up to your maximum weight, it's only that final set to failure that really counts.

The *work set* is a single set of six to eight repetitions to failure using a load equivalent to 75 to 80 percent of your 1RM. The load must be heavy enough for momentary muscular failure to be reached in six to eight repetitions. It is this final all-out effort during the work set that generates muscle overload and elicits hypertrophy. The only purpose of lighter warm-up sets in any given exercise is to prime your muscle to achieve one goal: a single all-out effort work set.

When you reach momentary muscular failure, squeezing out that last rep requires 100 percent intensity. But how can you be absolutely sure that *all* the muscle fibers have been recruited and that the muscle is totally exhausted? If you want to really annihilate the muscle, it's possible to go beyond failure and generate an even bigger hypertrophic response. Training beyond failure extends the work set into the zone of hyperintensity. This is an extreme stimulus that requires 110 percent effort. Even though the muscle has failed during the positive phase of the last rep, it is forced to perform more work. Later in this book, I describe 12 muscle-scorching steps to intensify your workouts (chapter 11).

To whet your appetite, here are three techniques to intensify your mass-building work set. First, when you hit failure during the positive (concentric) phase of the last rep, pause the weight in a static (isometric) contraction. Contract the muscle as hard as you can, and hold the weight as long as you can until you reach failure in the static contraction. Then lower the weight as slowly as possible, forcing those muscle fibers to perform a final negative (eccentric) contraction. Finally, get a training partner to assist you in performing one last forced repetition. This brutal assault takes place after your muscle reaches the point of positive failure. The muscle then fails during the static contraction and fails again during the negative phase. This is what beyond-failure training is all about—the set begins when the muscle fails.

Make no mistake: These methods of extending the set beyond the point of failure are intense. When used effectively, they produce the ultimate trigger for hypertrophic adaptation and incredible mass gains. The static contraction, the negative rep, and the forced rep are brutal tricks to go beyond failure and induce muscular overload. To avoid injury when training with this degree of intensity, you must have a spotter, especially if you're using free weights.

Rest Interval

An important variable for generating an overload effect in multiple-set training programs is the amount of rest allowed between sets. Muscle fibers experience physiological change only if they are both recruited and exhausted. If too much time passes between sets, the exhausted muscle fibers might recover and be used in the next set, thus training the same group of muscle fibers over and over.

The theory behind multiple sets is this: As long as the time between sets is not sufficient for the muscle fibers to recover from exhaustion, a different group of fibers will be recruited and overloaded during the next set. In this way, the multiple-set method might overload more muscle fibers and elicit greater adaptations than a one-set protocol.

The rest interval between sets must be specific, not random. Resting no more than two minutes results in more muscle fibers being overloaded.

Compare this system to shooting a gun. You take precise aim, making sure to hit the target with each shot. You deliver all six bullets, exhausting the gun of its firepower. Then you reload as quickly as possible to deliver the next round. Each set goes boom, boom, boom, with maximum precision and intensity.

The time taken between sets has an important relation to workout intensity. Power is the rate at which work is done. The quicker the work is performed, the more power is generated. In other words, your workout will be more intense when you complete it in less time. How much time you take to complete a workout naturally depends on the rest interval between sets. When your rest period is minimal, you complete the work in less time, and your workout is more intense. For a workout in which fat loss is a priority, shortening your rest interval is a useful way to burn more calories. An interval of 60 seconds or less allows just enough time to change the weight on the bar or relocate to the next exercise station.

Workout Time

Now we need to discuss the duration of your workout. This is based on your muscle's fuel tank—it is not an endless supply. Your muscle contains a store of chemical energy that is converted to mechanical energy. The muscle contracts, and movement occurs. Think of fuel stored in the gas tank of your vehicle. When burned, the chemical energy within gasoline is converted to mechanical energy. The wheels turn, and the vehicle moves along the road. When all the fuel is used up, the tank is empty, and your vehicle comes to a halt.

A similar process occurs inside your muscles. During exercise, your muscles' fuel tank begins to run low after 30 minutes; after an hour, it's empty. You are still able to exercise when your muscles' energy reserves are depleted because the muscles get energy from other sources in your body. But at this point, your muscles shift into an endurance mode, such as being put on cruise control. The problem is that you can no longer accelerate, so you can't achieve maximum muscle stimulus. Your muscles are merely surviving, not growing. If you venture into muscle cruise control, it will take days for your muscles to refill their fuel tank. Muscle building is an anaerobic process. The training stimulus should be short and intense, not long and steady. Do what's necessary to trigger the hypertrophic response, then leave the gym, go home, rest, and grow.

For muscle growth, your workout time should not exceed one hour. Ideally, you should be in and out of the gym within 30 to 45 minutes. Remember that after an hour you have lost your power. You're out of ammunition and are shooting blanks. Get out of the gym before it's too late.

Recovery

If your goal is muscle growth, the time that elapses between workouts for a given muscle group or body part is important. An intense workout in which sets are performed to the point of muscle failure represents a massive insult, causing ultrastructural damage and protein degradation within the muscle tissue. This degree of stress is necessary for muscle hypertrophy. During recovery, protein synthesis occurs at an increased rate inside the muscle cells, which results in a size increase in the muscle fibers during the repair process. Scientific studies indicate that it takes five to seven days of complete rest to repair the muscle fiber disruption.

During the recovery phase, the muscle should not participate in heavy resistance exercise that directly targets the same body part. If the muscle's repair process is interrupted by another heavy workout, it will not achieve its maximum growth potential. The recovering muscle is, however, capable of assisting with workouts for other body parts and participating in low-resistance aerobic exercise.

Fact or Fiction

Myth 1: Working out requires a huge time commitment.

False: With as few as three half-hour workouts each week, you can build bigger, stronger muscles and improve your health. That's a total time commitment of less than two hours a week. If your workout lasts more than an hour, you're probably overtraining. It's quality lifting that builds muscle, not quantity.

Myth 2: Lifting weights makes you muscle bound.

False: No matter how hard you hit the weights, you're not going to suddenly evolve into the Incredible Hulk. Your muscles will get bigger and stronger, but it's a gradual process that takes several months. Muscles can become a little stiff in response to exercise, so stretching is important to maintain flexibility.

Myth 3: All that muscle turns to fat if you stop lifting.

False: Muscle tissue cannot turn into fat—it's biologically impossible. Muscle is a protein structure filled with carbohydrate and water. Fat is a completely different molecule. It's like comparing metal and wood—not the same. Muscles get smaller if you quit lifting, but they won't morph into fat. However, if you stop exercising and continue to consume the same amount of food, the excess unused calories *will* make you fat.

To maximize muscle growth after an intense bout of hypertrophy training, the muscle should be rested for seven days. The ideal mass program should employ a split-training system in which each muscle group is trained once each week. Divide your body into sections to create a series of workouts that you repeat over a weekly cycle.

Split-training systems serve two valuable purposes. First, because the body is divided into sections, you get to focus all your efforts on a few selected muscle groups at each workout session. Second, even though you are performing several workouts per week, each individual muscle group is exercised only once every seven days, thereby allowing ample recovery time.

Time to Train

Scientific evidence suggests that the best time of day to train for *mass* may be the early evening, when the body tends to be strongest. On the flip side, the ideal time to train for *fat loss* might be first thing in the morning, when your body tends to burn body fat for fuel. The reality for most of us is that a workout must fit around our busy schedules. Ideally, you should be *consistent* with *when* you work out, whether it's first thing in the morning, on your lunch break, or after a long day at work. We are creatures of habit, and our bodies will perform better with a *regular* workout schedule. Your body will adapt, whatever time of day you train.

In this chapter you've learned the science behind muscle growth and how to manipulate the principles of weight training to create an effective workout. In the next chapter, we turn our attention from the gym and into the kitchen. Exercise is the spark, but nutrition provides the fuel for muscle growth and fat loss. Your diet dictates how your body responds to a workout, so read on to find out what to put in your mouth and when.

Feeding the Machine

It's true that we are what we eat. The problem is we eat too much. Food, glorious food, anytime, anywhere. Eating is so convenient that it's hard to resist gulping down more calories than we need. Please, sir, I want some more. Breakfast, brunch, lunch, then a munch on some snacks, followed by an appetizer, dinner, dessert, and around bedtime, a snack. It seems that during every waking hour, we're satisfying our cravings for delicious treats that dance on our taste buds.

Whereas the key factor in generating muscle mass is exercise, the secret ingredient in fat loss is diet. In other words, you can't build muscle unless you exercise. Even if you eat all those fancy supplements, your muscles won't grow if you don't exercise. On the other hand, nutrition plays the biggest role in losing body fat. With the right diet, you can lose weight, with or without exercise.

When it comes to providing fuel for your body, quality overrules quantity. You should be running on premium fuel. Your body works much better on the good stuff. If you want to build muscle and stay lean, proper nutrition is crucial.

But for many people, getting proper nutrition means dieting, and for some people dieting conjures up anxiety, fear, and loathing. One thing you'll be happy to hear is that my fuel prescription does not focus on food restriction. We pay more attention to other details, such as choice, preparation, and timing. You'll get to eat, all right—every three to four hours. But it's not going to be a burger, fries, and a soda.

HARD MUSCLE FUEL

You need six classes of nutrients to build and drive your human body: carbohydrate, protein, fat, vitamins, minerals, and water. The first three—carbohydrate, protein, and fat—are what we call macronutrients. They provide energy and structure to the body's cells and tissues. The other nutrients regulate body functions and the machinery inside our cells.

Water is the most critical element in the diet. Most of the other nutrients essential for life can function only in the presence of water. Under optimal conditions, the body can survive up to 60 days without food but no more than 10 days without water. During moderate activity levels under average environmental conditions, the body needs a gallon (or nearly 4 L) of water per day. Your muscles are made up of 60 to 70 percent water.

Calories are a measure of the energy value of food; they are the amount of energy you put into your body's fuel tank. If you consume more calories than you use during the course of each day, the excess energy is stored inside your body. In time, you'll gain weight. On the other hand, if you consume fewer calories than you need, you'll lose weight because your body burns fat stores in order to generate the extra energy requirement.

Designing your diet is easy, as long as you follow the steps of my hard muscle formula. It's important to remember that my fuel plan is not a starvation diet that involves an all-out restriction of food. The aim of this nutrition program is to provide nutrients to build muscle and encourage fat loss. You know that quick-fix starvation thing? Don't do it—it doesn't work.

The subtle changes we're going to make to your eating habits will melt away fat. Your nutrition program should be planned with intent; do not expect it to fall into place by accident. Although the process of designing your diet might seem tricky at first, it's not complicated. Once you get the hang of it, the process becomes simple. You can begin formulating your nutrition intake using the following steps. You may want a pen and paper to make your own calculations.

Step 1: Caloric Balance

The first step is to calculate your daily calorie requirement (DCR). This figure represents the amount of calories you need to perform daily activities. It's what I call the maintenance calorie requirement—the number of calories needed per day to maintain your current body weight. This simple calculation is made using the following formula:

$$\text{Body weight in pounds} \times 10 = \text{DCR}$$

$$\text{Body weight in kilograms} \times 22 = \text{DCR}$$

Let's say you weigh 180 pounds (82 kg). Your daily maintenance calorie requirement is 180×10, or 1,800 calories. Consume more than this amount per day, and you'll gain weight because your body is in a positive caloric balance. Eat fewer calories than this amount, and you'll lose weight because your body is in a negative caloric balance.

This calculation is a *rough* estimate of daily calorie intake for someone with a sedentary, nonphysical occupation. Remember that the amount of calories you use varies from day to day depending on your level of activity. If your goal is to lose body fat, your daily calorie intake should be 10 percent *less* than your maintenance requirement (e.g., for a 180-pound man, 1,800 minus 180 = 1,620 calories) so that you're in a negative caloric balance. If, on the other hand, your goal is to gain weight, your daily calorie intake should be 10 percent *more* that the maintenance value (e.g., 1,800 plus 180 = 1,980 calories) to ensure that you're in a positive caloric balance.

Step 2: Timing

The timing and spacing of your daily meals are important. You need to consider the number of meals consumed per day and the size of each meal. I recommend that you eat five or six small meals every three to four hours during the day rather than stuff yourself with the traditional triple feasts at breakfast, lunch, and dinner.

There are several reasons for this strategy. First, eating every few hours maintains a constant energy level. You won't feel lethargic between meals. Second, if you have extended gaps between meals, you become so hungry that you're tempted to overeat at the next sitting. The excess calories are likely stored as fat. Third, when you consume smaller meals, your stomach adapts by reducing in size. A smaller stomach requires less food to fill it, and you'll prevent that bloated-belly look. Finally, the amount of food your intestine can digest and absorb in one sitting is limited. For example, your gut is capable of extracting only 30 to 40 grams of protein from a single meal of solid food. If you consume larger meals, any excess nutrients may pass through without being absorbed, going to waste.

If you sleep 6 to 8 hours each night, that means you're awake for 16 to 18 hours during each 24-hour period. Fitting six meals into your day means eating every 2 to 3 hours. To calculate how many calories you need to consume at each meal to make up your daily calorie requirement, divide your DCR by 6. Go back to our example of the 180-pound person who requires 1,800 calories per day. When his DCR is divided by 6, it breaks down to 300 calories per meal. You see what I mean when I say you won't go hungry on this plan?

When planning your six daily meals, list them as meals 1 through 6, or, if you prefer tradition, call the meals breakfast, lunch, dinner, and supper, interspersed with nutritious midmorning and midafternoon snacks. You're allowed to juggle the calorie content of each meal as long as the total amount over the course of the

Empty Stomach: Is it better to train on an empty stomach?

Exercising and eating are two opposing biological situations, just like being asleep or awake. When you exercise, your body focuses on muscle function and switches off digestion in your gut. When you eat, the opposite happens: Your body focuses on digestion, diverting blood away from the muscles. In the fed state after a meal, the last thing your body wants to do is participate in vigorous exercise. In the fasting state when hungry, your body's hormonal balance is primed for action. Think about it: It's not easy to sleep when you're hungry, is it? So if you want to optimize athletic performance, it makes biological sense to exercise on an empty stomach, about two hours after your last meal.

day meets your daily calorie requirement. The diet plan for a 180-pound (82 kg) person doesn't have to be six 300-calorie meals. A person of that body weight might choose the following meal plan:

Breakfast: 300 calories

Midmorning snack: 150 calories

Lunch: 500 calories

Midafternoon snack: 150 calories

Dinner: 500 calories

Evening snack: 200 calories

Just make sure that your daily total—in this case, 1,800 calories—matches your daily requirement.

Step 3: Nutrients

The third step of the hard muscle formula is to adjust the relative proportion of nutrients that make up your daily intake of fuel. Coordinating the nutrient ratios in your diet is called food partitioning. I recommend a diet that is low in fat (especially saturated fat) and high in protein. The relative proportion of each nutrient in your diet is shown in table 2.1. The three dietary macronutrients that provide energy for your body are carbohydrate, protein, and fat. Not all nutrients are made equal, so the relative proportion of each is an important determinant of your overall calorie intake. Water and the dietary micronutrients (vitamins and minerals) do not directly contribute to your daily calorie intake, but they are essential components of a healthy diet.

Table 2.1 Macronutrient Ratios for Weight Gain and Weight Loss

Macronutrient	Weight gain	Weight loss
Protein	40%	50%
Carbohydrate	50%	40%
Fat	10%	10%
Calorie balance	Positive	Negative

Dietary fat (nine calories per gram) has more than twice the amount of calories per gram than protein or carbohydrate (four calories per gram). Why is this important? Well, let's say you want to consume 100 calories. You could have this amount by eating 11 grams of fat, but if you choose a protein or carbohydrate source, you'd get to eat 25 grams, twice the amount of food.

Dietary fat is relatively high in calories, so a diet that contains a lot of fat can amount to a large number of calories. In other words, for 100 calories you could eat a good-sized portion of tuna (protein) or brown rice (carbohydrate) but only a tiny chunk of cheese (fat). Your hunger will be better satisfied if your stomach is filled with tuna or rice rather than merely teased by a mouse-sized portion of cheese, right?

Protein

Proteins are large nitrogen-rich molecules made up of a long string of amino acids. Protein is a fundamental component of all living cells and is essential for the growth and repair of tissue. The term *protein* is derived from the Greek *proteios*, which means first. Protein provides the amino acid building blocks for muscle, and its high nitrogen content creates the right anabolic environment for muscle growth. When it comes to building muscle and losing body fat, protein is the king of all nutrients.

To build muscle, you need an adequate supply of raw materials. Sufficient protein is essential for building lean muscle mass. To get your fill, aim to consume 1 to 1.5 grams of protein per pound (.5 kg) of body weight. A person who weighs 180 pounds (82 kg) should try to eat at least 180 grams of protein each day. The DCR of a person weighing 180 pounds is 1,800 calories; if protein is to make up 50 percent of the DCR, he will need to consume the protein equivalent of 900 calories. To help meet this daily requirement, every meal should contain at least 30 grams of protein.

Daily protein intake = 1 to 1.5 grams per pound (.5 kg) of body weight

A high-protein diet is less likely to cause fat deposits than either a high-carbohydrate or high-fat diet. There are several reasons for this. First, many of the calories from protein are burned off during digestion through what is called the thermic effect of food. Of all the macronutrients, protein has the highest thermic effect; digestion burns off 25 percent of the calories consumed. In comparison, only 15 percent of the calories from carbohydrate are used during digestion. Fat has virtually no thermic effect. Second, unlike carbohydrate, protein does not stimulate a significant insulin response. Insulin, a storage hormone, neutralizes blood sugar and is responsible for depositing fat. Because the effect of protein on insulin secretion is negligible, the potential for fat storage is diminished. Third, protein consumption stimulates the secretion of glucagon, a hormone that opposes the effect of insulin. Since glucagon is a signal to burn fat for fuel, fat loss rather than fat gain tends to occur. So, the larger the protein component of your diet, the more effective are your powers of fat burning. There's no evidence that a high-protein diet has any detrimental effect on healthy people with normal kidney function, but it's recommended that a high-protein diet be accompanied by lots of fluids. Adequate liquid consumption—at least a gallon of water a day—helps flush your body of any protein by-products.

High-quality sources of dietary protein are beef, poultry, fish, egg whites, and milk. However, not all protein sources are created equal; some are better for building muscle than others. In fact, every protein source has a biological value (BV) that determines the quality of its protein content. The higher the BV, the better the protein is absorbed and used for muscle growth—in foods with higher BVs the protein is more bioavailable. So when it comes to choosing a protein source, pick the ones with the highest BV. The BVs of different protein sources are compared in table 2.2.

Table 2.2 Biological Values of Protein Sources

Protein source	Biological value (BV)
Whey protein	100+
Milk	100
Egg whites	88
Fish	83
Beef	80
Chicken	79
Soy	74

Table 2.3   Sources of Protein

Food sources of 30 g protein
1 6 oz (175 g) chicken breast
1 6 oz (175 g) turkey breast
6 oz (175 g) fish (e.g., tuna, salmon)
6 oz (175 g) lean beef
5 (large) egg whites
30 fluid oz (900 ml) nonfat milk

Selecting a portion of protein to accompany each meal is not difficult. Each portion should contain about 30 grams of protein. The amount of protein will of course vary depending on your individual requirement (based on body weight). The easiest way to check is to read the product label for a breakdown of its contents. For easy reference, use table 2.3 as a guide. Chapters 7, 10, and 14 also discuss individual protein requirements in more detail with the specific training programs.

Carbohydrate

Carbohydrates are sugar molecules and your body's preferred source of energy. Dietary carbohydrate is found in foods such as sugar, starch, and fiber. Carbohydrate comes in two forms: simple and complex.

Simple sugars (monosaccharides and disaccharides) such as glucose, fructose, and sucrose are found in cane sugar and fruits. Simple sugars are quick sources of energy. They have a high glycemic index (GI), which means they are absorbed quickly by the gut, causing a rapid increase in blood sugar.

Complex carbohydrates are larger polysaccharide molecules that provide a more sustained release of energy (lower GI). Complex carbohydrates include starch (potatoes, pasta, and rice) and fiber (vegetables, cereals, and whole grains). Dietary sources of carbohydrate with a lower GI are digested and absorbed slowly, maintaining a stable concentration of sugar in the blood.

The body converts carbohydrate into glucose for energy or into glycogen for energy storage in the liver and muscle. When glycogen stores are filled, excess carbohydrate is converted to fat. Even though dietary carbohydrate is essential for energy and muscle building, eating more carbohydrate than you need feeds your fat stores, inflating that spare tire around your waist.

Table 2.4   Sources of Carbohydrate

Food sources of 25 g carbohydrate*
1 oz (30 g) rice
1 oz (30 g) pasta
1.25 oz (40 g) oatmeal
1 medium potato
1 piece of fruit (e.g., banana, apple, orange)
8 fluid oz (240 ml) fruit juice

*Approximate values

High-quality sources of complex carbohydrate are brown rice, potatoes with the skin, whole-grain pasta, yams, oatmeal, and whole-wheat bread. Whole foods such as potatoes, yams, and fruits are types of carbohydrate that nature has portioned out for us. One medium-size potato is a single portion of carbohydrate to complement one of your daily meals. Table 2.4 itemizes single 25-gram portions of carbohydrate from a selection of dietary sources.

Remember that to partition your nutrient ratio of 50 percent protein to 40 percent carbohydrate (for weight loss), the portion of carbohydrate in each meal should be slightly less than that of protein. If you're shooting for 30 to 35 grams of protein per meal, the amount of carbohydrate should be about 25 to 30 grams.

Fruit   Fruits are high in vitamins, minerals, and fiber. That's the good news. The bad news is fruit contains the simple sugar fructose. Fructose produces a stable rise in blood sugar, but it has a downside for anyone trying to lose fat.

One problem is that fructose is readily converted into body fat. This means a proportion of the fruit you eat can ultimately end up as fat. What's more, high-fructose corn syrup is the main sweetener in soda. The regular consumption of soda has been linked to the rise in obesity rates. A second problem is that drinking juice or soda with a meal encourages fat uptake. Third, fructose does not efficiently restock the muscle's energy store of glycogen, which means you might not recover from your workouts effectively. After exercise, starchy and fibrous types of carbohydrate, such as that found in potatoes and whole-grain rice, restock more glycogen into the muscles—which promotes recovery—than does simple sugar. With just a fraction of simple sugar being converted to glycogen, the remaining will likely spill into fat stores.

To achieve that lean, muscular look, select complex carbohydrate foods instead of fruit. If you choose to get your daily dose of vitamins and minerals from fruit, that's okay, but remember—everything in moderation. By all means, choose your favorite piece of fruit. Bananas, oranges, apples, grapefruits, melons, peaches, strawberries, and blueberries are all very nutritious, but a single daily serving is all you need. Too much whole fruit or juice forms fat on the body. The diets outlined in this book typically include three portions of fruit or vegetables per day, in contrast to the general recommendation of five a day. Remember, this kind of public advice is aimed at those folk who don't exercise and live off a diet of burgers and fries. Furthermore, when you are following a calorie-controlled diet, it is difficult to calculate the exact nutrient content of a piece of fruit because it varies by size.

If you're aiming for that extremely ripped look by reducing your body fat to below 10 percent, you might notice a significant difference in your physique when you eliminate fruits and juices from your diet. Many competitive bodybuilders looking to get shredded don't include fruit in their precontest diets. If you choose to totally eliminate fruit from your diet for a short period, be sure to take a daily multivitamin and mineral supplement to prevent deficiency.

Fiber   Fiber, plant material resistant to digestion, is essential for proper digestion and prevents constipation. Dietary sources of fiber include bran, cereals, whole grains, vegetables, oatmeal, fruit, and brown rice. To keep your digestive tract running smoothly, the recommended daily intake of fiber is 25 grams.

Vegetables   Vegetables are healthy low-calorie foods. They are not a major source of carbohydrate or protein, but you should include a vegetable with two of your daily meals. Their primary benefits are that they are high in fiber and contain vitamins and antioxidants. They do you good! High-quality sources include broccoli, carrots, spinach, lettuce, tomatoes, cucumbers, green beans, squash, and cabbage. Buy your veggies fresh or frozen, not canned. Frozen veggies are convenient and just as nutritious as fresh. Serve them lightly steamed or raw.

Dietary Fat

Fats are molecules containing strings of fatty acids. In addition to being the body's alternative energy source to glucose, dietary fat has several important functions.

- Fat is an essential component of cell structure and nerves.
- The insulating layer of fat beneath the skin helps preserve body heat.
- Steroid hormones, including testosterone, are made from cholesterol.
- Fat is required to transport fat-soluble vitamins through the body.

Table 2.5 Dietary Fat Sources

Food source	Fat (g)
6 oz (175 g) lean beef	10
6 oz (175 g) salmon	8
6 oz (175 g) skinless chicken breast	6
1 whole egg	4
1.25 oz (40 g) oatmeal	3
6 oz (175 g) tuna fish (water packed)	2

Now don't forget that your body has plenty of stored fat already. What's more, your body is able to synthesize most of the fat it needs, with the exception of the essential fats such as the omega-3 and omega-6 fatty acids. Small amounts of unsaturated fat are essential in the diet because your body can't make them. So not all dietary fat is bad. Saturated fat, found in butter, animal fat, egg yolks, and lard, is the enemy. And trans fat (listed on food labels as hydrogenated vegetable oil) is the enemy as well. As a rule, you can identify bad fat because it's solid at room temperature. The healthier monounsaturated and polyunsaturated fats are liquid at room temperature. Examples of unsaturated fat sources are olive oil, flaxseed oil, canola oil, fish oil, sesame oil, safflower oil, and nuts. Too much fat (just as too much of any nutrient) is unhealthy, period. It leads to obesity, diabetes, and an increased risk of heart disease. Excess saturated fat raises LDL (bad) cholesterol and lowers HDL (good) cholesterol. The result is clogged arteries, high blood pressure, and heart attacks. You certainly shouldn't be concerned with *adding* fat to your diet. Even with the best efforts to eliminate fat, the stuff finds its way into your diet. As you can see in table 2.5, small amounts of fat are in many of the foods we eat.

The nutritionally essential fatty acids are omega-3 (e.g., linolenic acid) and omega-6 (e.g., linoleic acid). These fats are important for cardiovascular health and immune function. Dietary sources of omega-3 and omega-6 fatty acids are salmon, nuts, eggs, avocado, cereals, and flaxseed and linseed oil. If you wish to ensure a daily supply of these essential fats, the simplest solution is to supplement with flaxseed or linseed oil or a fish oil gel capsule.

The recommended daily intake of fat is 20 percent of your total calories. But if you want to ditch that spare tire, aim to keep your fat intake around 10 percent, which amounts to 15 to 20 grams a day. Even when you try diligently to restrict your fat intake, at the end of the day, it'll probably creep up toward 20 percent without your realizing it. If you want to add some healthy polyunsaturated fat to your diet, use a tablespoon of flaxseed or canola oil mixed with vinegar as a salad dressing. Alternatively, a few servings of fish each week provide adequate amounts of good fat.

Vitamins and Minerals

Vitamins and minerals are essential dietary micronutrients. They serve many functions in the body, and dietary deficiency can result in ill health. Although these micronutrients don't themselves enhance athletic performance, they're necessary to achieve optimal levels of performance.

A well-balanced diet provides all the essential vitamins and minerals. But if you're involved in an intense exercise program, you'll require additional amounts of certain micronutrients. The simple solution to avoid deficiency is to take a daily multivitamin and mineral supplement. You have enough dietary concerns without worrying about individual vitamin or mineral consumption. If you pay too much

> ## Postworkout: After a workout, should I eat solid food or drink a liquid meal?
>
> Heavy resistance exercise degrades muscle protein and depletes muscle glycogen. As part of the muscle's anabolic response to exercise, muscle protein synthesis and glycogen resynthesis begin immediately. And the sooner you provide the necessary building blocks of protein and carbohydrate, the quicker the muscle repairs the protein damage and restocks its glycogen energy store. Immediately after your workout, your body is a sponge for soaking up nutrients, so there is a window of anabolic opportunity. Scientific study has shown that if you consume protein and carbohydrate immediately after training, you can gain more muscle mass than if you wait an hour or two after the workout. To take advantage of that nutrition window of growth, you'll need quick-acting liquid nutrients rather than a solid meal that sits in your stomach for several hours. The best way to produce a potent anabolic effect is to drink a protein and carbohydrate supplement within 30 minutes of your workout. What's more, drinking liquid after you work out is essential for rehydrating and replenishing body fluids. Remember that a well-hydrated muscle is an anabolic muscle! Because your muscles consist of around 70 percent water, maintaining your body's hydration ensures maximum muscle cell volume and promotes muscular growth.

attention to these micronutrients, you might miss the bigger picture. Nevertheless, a few micronutrients, such as calcium and vitamins B, C, and E, deserve a brief discussion for those participating in regular exercise.

Calcium is essential for strong bones; the recommended daily intake is 1,000 to 1,200 mg. The B-complex family of vitamins is important for metabolism and energy production. Vitamin C has an important role in postexercise recovery in that it's needed for the synthesis of collagen and the repair of tissues, such as muscle and tendons. Vitamin C might also minimize delayed-onset muscle soreness after exercise. Because many athletes have suboptimal levels of vitamin C, supplementing the diet with 500 to 1,000 mg per day might enhance overall performance. Both vitamins C and E are powerful antioxidants. Vitamin E protects against harmful free radicals generated during exercise and thereby boosts immunity. Beneficial effects are obtained with daily doses of 400 international units (IUs).

Water

Last but not least on the list of essential nutrients is water. Your body is 60 to 70 percent water, and good old H_2O is essential for life. Remember to consume at least a gallon (nearly 4 L) of water a day. Unlike most other thirst quenchers, water is calorie free.

PLANNING MEALS

Selecting the content of your diet is easy. You can create six healthy meals each day by using the food chart in table 2.6.

Choose a portion of protein and carbohydrate from each section to make a meal. Add a serving of vegetables to at least two of your daily meals. Healthy vegetable choices include carrots, broccoli, spinach, green beans, peas, lettuce, tomato, cucumber, green pepper, and celery.

You need to eat clean to be lean. If your diet consists of "clean" food, you reduce the chance of consuming hidden calories that appear during food preparation or as flavoring. Try to avoid using cooking fats or oils. Eat sauces, marinades, and food dressings sparingly. These seemingly innocent additions can significantly bump up the calorie count of your meal by adding extra fat and carbohydrate. For instance, a single serving of sauce, margarine spread, or marinade contains 40 calories or more. If you need to add some flavor, try a tablespoon of ketchup or mustard, which contains only 15 calories of carbohydrate. Alternatively, try adding some spices (see page 24).

I'll remind you again here to think before you drink. A glass of most beverages, including soda, juice, beer, or wine, contains 100 calories or more. When possible, drink water.

As you gain experience in creating nutritious meals, you can take a calorie count and compare it to your daily requirement calculation. Reading product labels is the best way to go. If the food is clean, it's easier to approximate your calorie intake. Use a calculator to figure out how your daily intake of nutrients matches up to the protein, carbohydrate, fat split of 50-40-10. Adjust your eating as necessary.

Table 2.6 Food Choices

	Food sources
Protein	Skinless chicken breast
	Turkey breast, lean ground turkey
	Salmon, water-packed tuna
	Lean ground beef, top sirloin steak, top round steak
	Egg whites
	Lean ham
	Low-fat or nonfat cottage cheese
	Low-fat or nonfat yogurt
	Hard cheeses*
	Nuts*
	Edamame/soy nuts*
	Tofu*
Carbohydrate	Whole-grain rice, whole-grain pasta
	Potato, yam
	Oatmeal, whole-wheat bread
	Orange, apple, banana, melon, grapefruit

*These foods may contain high amounts of fat. Check their nutrition facts.

Finally, remember that your daily meal schedule will need to accommodate your workout. It doesn't matter what time of day you train because the core energy inside your muscles comes from the food you ate the day before.

PREPARATION

Preparing your meals is straightforward, but following a few simple rules can't hurt. You may also want to abandon or take a critical look at some of your old cooking habits. The key principle in preparation is to avoid adding additional calories, particularly from fat.

Solid meats, such as chicken, turkey breast, fish, and steak, can be grilled, baked, or broiled. Squeeze some lemon juice over the meat, or lightly paste it with a low-fat marinade. Don't forget to remove the skin from chicken and turkey (or use skinless cuts). Don't deep fry meat or smother it with butter or high-fat sauce. Lean ground beef or turkey can be fried in a nonstick pan. Drain off any fat or water accumulated during cooking. If you really want to clean the meat, put the cooked meat into a sieve, rinse it with water, and then reheat it before serving.

Egg whites can be scrambled in a nonstick pan with or without a nonfat cooking spray. Crack open the egg and remove the yolk. Each egg white contains 6 grams of protein, so you'll need five or six large eggs to get enough protein for a meal. Add one half or one whole yolk, if you wish. Cook eggs until dry to reduce the risk of salmonella bacterial poisoning.

Other sources of protein, such as water-packed tuna or low-fat cottage cheese, don't require any preparation.

For carbohydrate, potatoes can be baked, boiled, or cooked in a microwave oven. Don't add butter or sour cream. Steam your rice. Boil your pasta. Check food labels to calculate a 25- to 30-gram portion of carbohydrate. Eat the pasta plain or squeeze a lemon over it. Don't use sauce, butter, or cheese. A portion of whole-wheat bread is usually two slices. Remember that if you use a low-fat spread, you'll add about 50 calories from fat.

Early Bird Workout

If you train in the morning, your core energy comes from what you ate the day before. You should not eat any solid food within two hours of working out. Nevertheless, here are some simple steps you can take to aid performance and recovery:

1. Upon waking, rehydrate with water.
2. Boost your blood glucose with a glass of orange juice.
3. Drink a cup of coffee if you want an extra kick start.
4. Hydrate regularly during your workout.
5. After your workout, grab a liquid protein and carbohydrate drink.
6. A dose of creatine and glutamine may also enhance recovery.

Add a portion of vegetables to at least two of your daily meals. They are an excellent source of vitamins and dietary fiber. Serve them lightly steamed or raw; don't cook them in butter. If you require a salad dressing, mix a tablespoon of healthy unsaturated oil such as safflower or olive with some vinegar.

Any nutrition program needs planning. If you don't have the appropriate foods available when and where you need them, you'll have a tough time sticking to your diet. If your kitchen is not stocked with the right food, you'll end up eating the wrong food. Planning your meals starts with making a detailed list before you visit the grocery store. Another tip: Don't go to the grocery store hungry. A hungry mind is less disciplined. Stick to the items on your list. Stock up on quality. If it's not on your list of healthy foods, don't buy it. Don't even look at it. When your house is free of junk food, you won't succumb to a damaging snack attack. When it comes to avoiding junk food, "out of sight, out of mind" is the best policy.

SPICE UP YOUR DIET

Herbs and spices can make your food taste better without adding significant amounts of extra calories. One teaspoon of the following spices contains five calories or less, with zero fat and zero carbohydrate. What's more, some of these taste enhancers have additional benefits for body sculpting beyond flavor. Here are some ingredients that can spice up your physique.

- **Garlic** has been linked to combating everything from cancer and heart disease to the common cold. It also increases testosterone production and blunts the stress hormone cortisol. The result is higher testosterone levels, with a slight anabolic advantage for bigger muscles.
- **Ginger** is known to be good for settling stomach upset and fighting inflammation. But it has also been shown to increase fat burning by raising metabolism. This benefit has been demonstrated with both fresh and dried ginger, so take your pick.
- **Cinnamon** has been used as an antifungal agent and to ease indigestion, but it may also help muscle cells take in more of the insulin in your bloodstream. This increases the uptake of amino acids, creatine, and other nutrients into muscle tissue, thereby boosting growth.
- **Cayenne pepper** not only gives a kick to your taste buds but also can boost your metabolism. This spice contains a phytochemical that can increase metabolism and also reduce appetite—useful if you are looking to lose body fat.

ENJOY A CHEAT DAY

Sticking to your diet requires discipline. With all that choice out there, restricting your intake can lead to cravings, and these cravings can drive you crazy. With this in mind, I'm granting you permission to cut yourself some slack. I recommend that you take one cheat day per week. On your cheat day, you can eat whatever you want. Be that kid in a candy store. Get those cravings out of your system.

Your cheat day can be any day of the week. You might choose Sunday or a day that coincides with a particular social occasion, such as a dinner party, birthday, or other gathering. Whatever day you pick, make the most of it. It won't hurt to pig out one day a week—it's the long-term dietary discipline that counts.

Dining out at cafés or restaurants is best done on your free day because you have little if any control over the calorie content of meals prepared by other people. Your cheat day also allows you to balance your diet by including nutrients you would otherwise restrict, such as healthy fats and fruit juices.

MODIFICATION

The hard muscle formula outlined in this chapter should serve as a blueprint. The calculations are a guide; nothing is carved in stone. We all metabolize foods in different ways. Just as each of us has a different body type, individual results from any nutrition program will vary. To accommodate individual variation, the blueprint might need to be modified. Your own food portions will depend on your daily calorie allowance, which in turn depends on your body weight and your daily calorie expenditure. The quantity of food in each of your daily meals will also depend on your goal—do you want to gain weight or lose weight?

If you're a lean ectomorph who wants to gain weight, you should consume additional calories in the form of carbohydrate. In such a case, the nutrient ratio should approximate that recommended in the mass generator program—50 percent carbohydrate, 40 percent protein, and 10 percent fat. On the other hand, if you're an endomorph who needs to cut back on carbohydrate to lose weight, you should follow the body fat blitz program: 50 percent protein, 40 percent carbohydrate, and 10 percent fat. Chapter 4 further discusses body types. To coordinate your own requirements, chart your progress each month, and then adjust your daily calorie intake and carbohydrate consumption as necessary. Increase your intake for additional weight gain, and decrease your intake for additional weight loss. However, whenever you modify your diet, do so in *small* stepwise increments. If you add too many calories too soon, you'll risk gaining fat instead of lean muscle. Likewise, if you cut back on too many calories too soon, you'll risk losing muscle mass as well as body fat.

Remember that it's overconsumption of calories that causes unhealthy weight gain. No matter what you eat, if it has calories and you consume too much of it, you'll end up gaining weight.

In body sculpting, the challenge is to provide the right nutrients to fuel muscle growth and burn body fat. In this chapter you've learned the key components you need to feed your body. Later in the book, I show how to combine these ingredients to cook up winning recipes to generate muscle mass and blitz body fat.

Meet the Muscles

Heads may turn at the sight of bulging biceps, but jaws drop in the presence of sculpted bodywork. And the key to building a jaw-dropping, custom-built body is to know your anatomy. When you think about it, changing the way your body looks means modifying your anatomy. Muscular proportion and symmetry are created by intelligent exercise choices and not by chance. You should skillfully use weights to sculpt your body, not just to indiscriminately pack on pounds of flesh. So don't gamble with your training. Walk into the gym with a winning strategy. By taking the guesswork out of body sculpting, your efforts at the gym will be more productive. When you know your anatomy, you'll be able to customize your body with clinical precision. So let's peel back the skin and reveal the muscles you'll be working with. Figure 3.1 is a whole-body picture of what muscles lie beneath the surface.

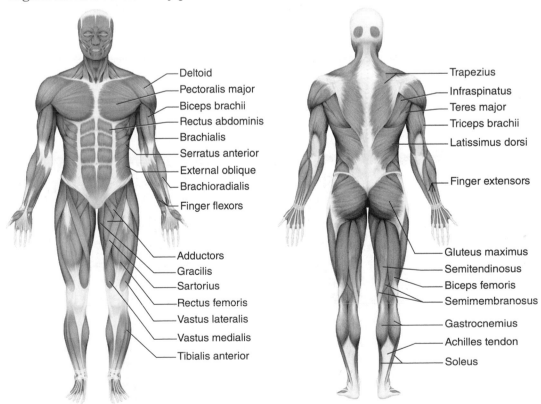

Figure 3.1 Front and rear view of full body.

CHEST

The *pectoralis major* is a fan-shaped muscle that has two anatomic sections, or heads (figure 3.2). The upper *clavicular* head arises from the clavicle (collarbone), and the lower *sternal* head arises from the sternum (breastbone). The two heads pass outward across the chest wall and merge into a single tendon that attaches to the humerus bone in the upper arm. As the muscle inserts, the tendon twists so that the upper head attaches beneath the lower head. When the pectoralis muscle contracts, movement takes place at the shoulder joint. Pectoralis major adducts, flexes, and internally rotates the arm, thus moving the arm forward and across the chest during movements such as push-ups or a bear hug. Even though the muscle has only two anatomic divisions, functionally it may be considered in three sections (upper, middle, and lower) depending on the angle through which the arm is moved. As the position of the shoulder joint changes, certain fibers of the chest muscle have a better mechanical advantage to create motion. Other fibers of the chest muscle are still active but are not able to contract as much because of shoulder position.

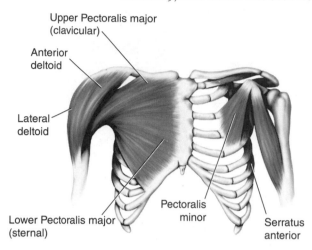

Figure 3.2 Anatomy of the chest and shoulder.

Upper Pectoralis major (clavicular)

Anterior deltoid

Lateral deltoid

Lower Pectoralis major (sternal)

Pectoralis minor

Serratus anterior

The *serratus anterior* muscle forms part of the sidewall of the chest. This muscle arises from the scapula behind and passes forward around the chest wall to attach to the upper eight ribs. The serrated edge of this muscle emerges from beneath the outer margin of the pectoralis muscle, sending fingerlike projections into the external oblique. Serratus anterior pulls (or protracts) the scapula forward, stabilizing the scapula against the chest wall. The serratus anterior provides an essential accessory function whenever the pectoralis major and latissimus dorsi muscles contract. It can also be targeted during exercises that work the abdominal oblique muscles.

Table 3.1 provides a list of exercises that target the chest muscles.

Table 3.1 Chest Exercises

Upper chest	Midchest	Lower chest
Incline barbell press	Barbell bench press	Decline press
Incline dumbbell press	Dumbbell bench press	Decline dumbbell fly
Incline dumbbell fly	Dumbbell fly	Cable crossover
Low-pulley cable fly	Machine fly	Chest dip

SHOULDERS

The shoulder is a ball-and-socket joint between the humerus bone of the upper arm and the scapula bone (shoulder blade). Six main movements occur at the shoulder: flexion, extension, abduction, adduction, internal rotation, and external rotation. During shoulder flexion, the upper arm is elevated forward toward the face. During shoulder extension, the arm moves backward behind the plane of the body. During abduction, the arm moves up and out to the side of the body. During adduction, the arm is pulled in toward the side of the body. Horizontal abduction and adduction occur when the arm moves in a horizontal plane at shoulder level, such as during chest flys or rear deltoid flys.

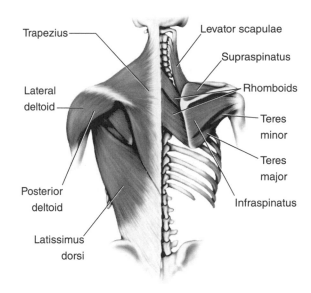

The *deltoid* muscle of the shoulder consists of three separate sections, or *heads*, each capable of moving the arm in different directions (figure 3.3). From a broad tendon attachment above the shoulder joint, the deltoid's three heads merge into a single tendon that attaches to the humerus bone of the upper arm. *Anterior* deltoid in front attaches to the clavicle and raises the arm forward. *Lateral* deltoid at the side attaches to the acromion and lifts the arm outward. *Posterior* deltoid behind attaches to the scapula and moves the arm backward.

Figure 3.3 Anatomy of the shoulder and back: rear view.

The *rotator cuff* is a group of four muscles that form a protective sleeve around the shoulder joint (figure 3.4). Despite being a barely visible muscle group, the rotator cuff is essential for shoulder stability and strength. All four muscles originate from the scapula (shoulder blade) and pass across the shoulder joint to attach onto the humerus bone of the upper arm. *Supraspinatus* lies above the joint and functions to raise (abduct) the arm up and outward—as for hailing a taxi. *Infraspinatus* and *teres minor* are located behind and act to rotate the arm out—as for hitchhiking. *Subscapularis* is situated in front and functions to rotate the arm inward—as for folding your arms across the chest.

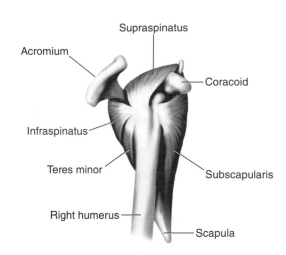

Table 3.2 provides a list of exercises that target the muscles of the shoulder.

Figure 3.4 Anatomy of the rotator cuff: side view.

Table 3.2 Shoulder Exercises

Front deltoid	Side deltoid	Rear deltoid	Rotator cuff
Barbell shoulder press	Dumbbell lateral raise	Bent-over dumbbell raise	External rotation
Dumbbell shoulder press	Cable lateral raise	Bent-over cable raise	Internal rotation
Dumbbell front raise	Machine lateral raise	Reverse cable crossover	Inclined side raise
Barbell front raise	Barbell upright row	Machine rear deltoid fly	Cable lateral raise
Cable front raise			

BACK

Anatomically, the rear torso, or back, consists of several layers of muscle, stacked like a sandwich. Functionally, and for bodybuilding purposes, the back is best considered in three sections, resembling triangular segments of a quilted blanket. Note that trapezius and latissimus dorsi are concerned primarily with movements of the shoulder and arm. (See figure 3.3 on page 29.) It is the erector spinae muscles that cause movements of the back and torso.

1. Upper back: The upper back is made up of a large triangular-shaped muscle called *trapezius*, which originates along the upper spine from the skull down to the last rib (i.e., all the cervical and thoracic vertebrae). The *upper* fibers of trapezius (in the neck) attach to the outer tip of the shoulder on the clavicle, acromion, and scapula. The *lower* fibers of trapezius (in the upper back) attach to the scapula (or shoulder blade). The upper traps provide support to the shoulders and are used to shrug the shoulders. The lower traps retract the scapula and pull the shoulders backward. Underneath the trapezius are three muscles that anchor the scapula to the spine: the levator scapulae, rhomboid major, and rhomboid minor. The rhomboid muscles work with the lower traps to retract the scapula. These so-called scapular retractor muscles lie under the trapezius and add muscular thickness to the upper back.

2. Middle back: *Latissimus dorsi* is a large fan-shaped muscle that arises from the lower half of the spinal column and the rear ridge of the pelvic bone (posterior iliac crest). From its large origin, the latissimus converges into a bandlike tendon that attaches to the upper humerus (next to the tendon of pectoralis major). The latissimus dorsi pulls the upper arm downward and backward (shoulder extension); hence, this muscle is targeted by pull-downs, pull-ups, and rows. The latissimus also pulls the arm in against the side of the body (adduction).

3. Lower back: The lower section is made up of the *erector spinae* (or *sacrospinalis*) muscles that run alongside the entire length of the spinal column. In the lumbar region, the erector spinae splits into three columns, namely *iliocostalis*, *longissimus*, and *spinalis*. These muscles are the pillars of strength in the lower back that keep the spine straight and *extend* the torso, arching the spine backward.

Table 3.3 provides a list of exercises that target the muscles of the back.

Table 3.3 Back Exercises

Upper back (trapezius)	Latissimus dorsi	Lower back
Barbell shrug	Wide-grip pull-down	Lumbar extension
Dumbbell shrug	Close-grip pull-down	Deadlift
Barbell upright row	Barbell row	Good morning lift
Seated cable row	Dumbbell row	
Chin-up	Machine row	

ARMS

Biceps: As its name suggests, the *biceps* muscle has two heads (figure 3.5). The *short head* attaches to the coracoid process, and the *long head* arises from above the glenoid of the shoulder joint. The two-headed muscle passes down alongside the humerus and attaches about 1.5 inches (4 cm) below the elbow joint onto a tuberosity on the inside of the radius bone. The biceps causes *flexion* at the elbow joint (i.e., raising the hand toward the face). The biceps also causes *supination* of the forearm (i.e., rotating the hand so the palm faces upward, the "get change" position).

In addition to the biceps, two other muscles *flex* (or bend) the elbow, namely the *brachialis* and *brachioradialis*. The brachialis muscle lies deep under the biceps, arising from the lower half of the humerus and attaching to the ulna bone just below the elbow joint. So, the *brachialis* lifts the *ulna* at the same time that the *biceps* lifts the *radius*. The brachioradialis muscle arises from the outer aspect of the lower end of the humerus then travels down the forearm to attach to the radius just above the wrist joint.

Triceps: The *triceps* muscle possesses three heads, or sections (figure 3.6). The *long head* arises from beneath the glenoid fossa of the shoulder joint, the *lateral (outer) head* from the outer surface of the humerus, and the *medial (inner) head* from the medial and rear surface of the humerus. All three heads fuse at their lower ends to form a single tendon that attaches behind the elbow joint onto the olecranon process of the ulna bone. The triceps causes *extension* at the elbow (i.e., moving the hand away from the face). The triceps is the only muscle that straightens the elbow joint, whereas three muscles (biceps, brachialis, and brachioradialis) bend the elbow. All three heads of the triceps muscle cross the elbow joint, but the *long head* also crosses beneath the shoulder joint.

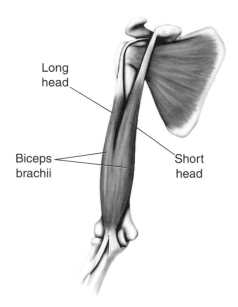

Figure 3.5 Anatomy of the biceps.

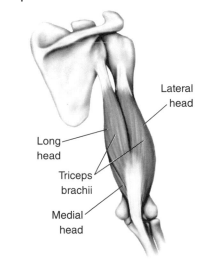

Figure 3.6 Anatomy of the triceps.

Forearm: The forearm is a mass of some 20 different muscles. It has two separate muscle compartments, the *flexor* group on the palm side (figure 3.7) and the *extensor* group on the reverse side (figure 3.8). The fleshy muscle portions of almost all these muscles are located in the upper two-thirds of the forearm. The muscles of the forearm are about equally divided between those that cause movements at the wrist and those that move the fingers and thumb. *Supination*, rotating the hand so the palm faces up ("get change"), is performed by the *supinator* and *biceps*. *Pronation*, rotating the hand so the palm faces down ("give change"), is performed by the *pronator teres* and *pronator quadratus*.

Other forearm muscles include the wrist flexors (palmaris longus, flexor carpi radialis, flexor carpi ulnaris); finger flexors (flexor digitorum superficialis, flexor digitorum profundus, flexor pollicis longus); wrist extensors (extensor carpi radialis longus and brevis, extensor carpi ulnaris); and finger extensors (extensor digitorum, extensor pollicis longus and brevis, extensor indicis).

Table 3.4 provides a list of exercises that target the arm muscles.

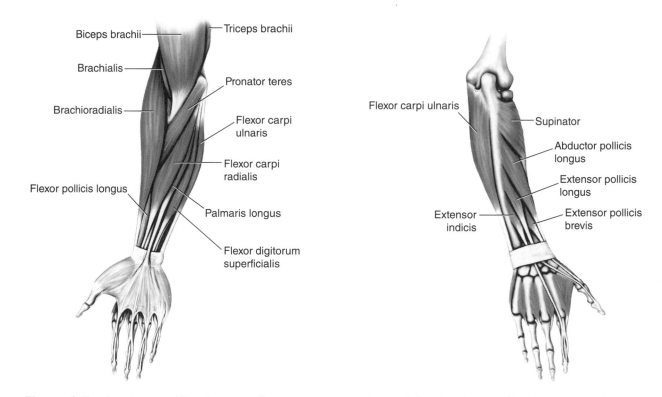

Figure 3.7 Anatomy of the forearm flexors.

Figure 3.8 Anatomy of the forearm extensors.

Table 3.4 Arm Exercises

Biceps	Triceps	Forearms
Barbell curl	Triceps push-down	Wrist curl
Dumbbell curl	Triceps dip	Reverse wrist curl
Concentration curl	Lying triceps extension	Reverse barbell curl
Cable curl	Seated triceps press	Hammer curl
Preacher curl	Close-grip bench press	
Machine curl	Dumbbell kickback	

LEGS

Your leg is divided into the upper leg (thigh) (figures 3.9 and 3.10) and lower leg (calf) (figure 3.11). The upper leg consists of one bone, the femur, whereas the lower leg consists of two bones, the tibia (on the big-toe side) and fibula (on the little-toe side). The knee is a hinge joint formed at the junction between the femur and the tibia. Two movements occur at the knee joint: flexion and extension. During knee flexion, the lower leg bends toward the back of the thigh. During knee extension, the lower leg moves away from the thigh so the leg becomes straight. The hip is a ball-and-socket joint between the upper end of the femur and the pelvic bone. Six main movements occur at the hip joint: flexion, extension, abduction, adduction, internal rotation, and external rotation. During hip flexion, the thigh bends up toward the abdomen, while during hip extension, the thigh moves backward to the rear. Your thighs separate during hip abduction and come together during hip adduction. The ankle is a hinge joint between the lower tibia and fibula and the talus bone in the foot. During ankle dorsiflexion, your toes lift off the ground, and the foot moves toward your shin. During ankle plantar flexion, your heel lifts off the floor, and the foot moves away from your shin.

Quadriceps femoris: The *quadriceps* in the front of the thigh has four separate heads: (1) *Rectus femoris* arises from the front of the pelvic bone; (2) *vastus medialis* arises from the inner edge of the femur bone; (3) *vastus lateralis* arises from the outer edge of the femur; (4) and *vastus intermedius* arises from the

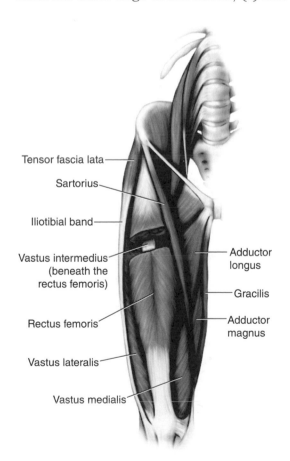

Figure 3.9 Anatomy of the thigh muscles: front view.

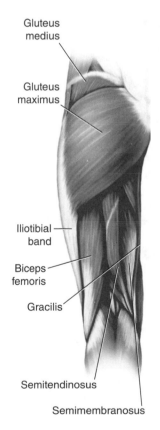

Figure 3.10 Anatomy of the leg: rear view.

front surface of the femur and lies underneath rectus femoris. The four heads merge together, attach onto the patella (kneecap), and then insert via a single (patellar) tendon onto the tibia, just below the knee joint. The main function of the quadriceps is to extend the knee and straighten the leg. Because the rectus femoris arises from the pelvic bone, contraction of this muscle also flexes the hip joint.

Hamstrings: The *hamstrings*, located behind the thigh, are a group of three muscles that all originate from the ischium bone of the pelvis. *Biceps femoris* passes behind the outer aspect of the thigh to attach to the head of the fibula bone, just below the knee; *semimembranosus* and *semitendinosus* pass together behind the inner aspect of the thigh, attaching to the upper tibia bone. All three hamstrings span both the knee and hip joints. Therefore they serve dual functions, causing flexion of the knee and extension of the hip.

Gluteals: *Gluteus maximus* arises from the large area on the rear of the pelvic bone, passes down behind the hip joint, and attaches onto the upper femur. This powerful muscle causes hip extension.

Other thigh muscles include the hip adductors (inner thigh) (gracilis, adductor longus, adductor magnus, adductor brevis); hip abductors (tensor fasciae latae, gluteus medius, gluteus minimus); and hip flexors (sartorius, iliopsoas, rectus femoris).

Calves: The lower leg contains 10 different muscles (figure 3.11). The calf comprises two muscles: *Gastrocnemius* is the visible muscle of the calf. The two heads (medial and lateral) of gastrocnemius arise from the rear of the femur bone, immediately above the knee joint. *Soleus* arises from the rear aspect of the tibia and lies underneath the gastrocnemius. The tendons of gastrocnemius and soleus fuse to form the Achilles tendon, which passes behind the ankle joint and attaches to the calcaneus (heel bone). The calf muscles cause plantar flexion of the ankle, the movement required to stand on tiptoes. The relative contribution of the two calf muscles depends on the angle of knee flexion. Gastrocnemius is the prime mover when the leg is straight, and soleus becomes more active as the knee bends. Note that gastrocnemius crosses both the knee and ankle joints and therefore serves a double function, causing knee flexion and ankle flexion.

Other lower leg muscles include *tibialis anterior* (ankle extension); *tibialis posterior* (ankle inversion); *peroneus longus* and *peroneus brevis* (ankle eversion); and the toe flexors and extensors (*flexor digitorum longus, flexor hallucis longus, extensor digitorum longus, extensor hallucis longus*).

Table 3.5 provides a list of exercises that target the leg muscles.

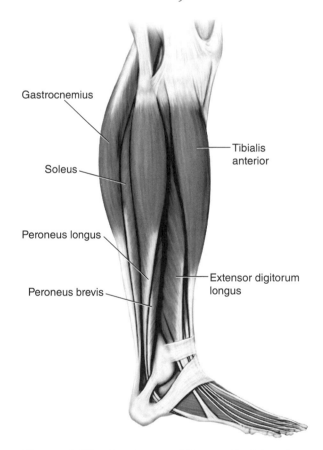

Gastrocnemius

Soleus

Peroneus longus

Peroneus brevis

Tibialis anterior

Extensor digitorum longus

Figure 3.11 Anatomy of the calf: side view.

Table 3.5 Leg Exercises

Quadriceps	Hamstrings	Rear deltoid	Rotator cuff
Leg extension	Lying leg curl	Cable kickback	Standing calf raise
Barbell squat	Standing leg curl	Hip extension	Seated calf raise
Leg press	Stiff-leg deadlift		Machine calf raise
Hack squat			Donkey calf raise
Lunge			

ABDOMINALS

The abdominal wall can be divided into two separate anatomic parts, each of which functions differently (figure 3.12). The *front wall* consists of one muscle, the *rectus abdominis*, (a.k.a. the abs). This muscle arises from the lower margin of the rib cage and sternum and passes vertically downward to attach on the pubic bone. The two rectus abdominis muscles (one on each side) are encased in a sheath of fascia that forms the central demarcation down the middle of the abs, known as the *linea alba*. Fascia divisions in the muscles are responsible for the "six-pack" appearance. The rectus muscles cause flexion of the trunk (i.e., bending the torso forward toward the legs). The motion is carried out by the *upper* abs pulling the rib cage down toward the pelvis or by the *lower* abs lifting the pelvis upward toward the chest.

The *sidewall* consists of three layers of muscles. The *external oblique* is the outer visible layer that passes obliquely downward from the rib cage to the pelvic bone. The middle layer, the *internal oblique*, passes obliquely upward from the pelvic bone to the ribs. Internal oblique lies under external oblique, and the fibers of the two muscles pass at right angles to one another. The innermost layer is the *transversus abdominis*, which lies horizontally across the abdominal wall. Contraction of the oblique muscles on one side causes the torso to bend sideways. Contraction of the obliques simultaneously on both sides assists the rectus muscle in flexing the trunk and also functions to splint the abdominal wall whenever a weight is lifted. Note that only the outer external oblique is visible.

Table 3.6 provides a list of exercises that target the abdominal muscles.

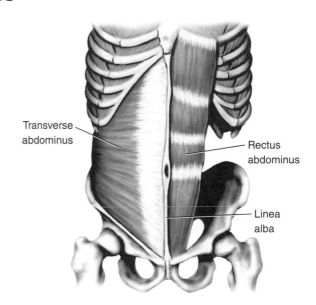

Transverse abdominus

Rectus abdominus

Linea alba

Figure 3.12 Anatomy of the abdominal wall.

Table 3.6 Abdominal Exercises

Upper abs	Lower abs	Sidewall obliques
Sit-up	Vertical leg raise	Twisting sit-up
Crunch	Incline leg raise	Oblique crunch
Rope crunch	Bench leg raise	Cable side crunch
Machine crunch	Reverse crunch	Dumbbell side bend
Decline sit-up		Dumbbell pullover
		Broomstick twist

The key to customizing your body is building muscle in the right places using a strategic selection of the best exercises. Now that you know your anatomy, your efforts in the gym will be more productive. In the next chapter, you'll learn how to choose the best body-sculpting program for your own individual goals.

Program Prescription

Attention, all readers! *There is no single method that suits every individual body type.* So before you begin, you must read this chapter. The objective is to help you choose the program that's right for you. Consider this: Everyone who walks into a supermarket has a different shopping list, right? You wouldn't go to the store with someone else's list, would you? Nope, you need to compile your own list to include everything you need. And to make this list, you've got to prepare beforehand by asking certain key questions. For example, do you need eggs, and if so how many? So when it comes to body sculpting, you must address the key issues. What's your body type? Is your main goal to gain muscle or lose body fat? How much gym time and workout experience do you have? And so on.

IDENTIFYING YOUR BODY TYPE

We have different body types, just as we have different personalities. Your body is as individual as your fingerprints. The way you look is determined much more by your genes—the information contained in your body's cells—than by the jeans you're wearing. The key to creating your own workout program lies in understanding body types and building a regimen that accommodates your unique form rather than trying to change it. If you customize exercise and diet to your own specific body type, you'll achieve a more effective transformation.

The three basic body types are ectomorph, mesomorph, and endomorph. An ectomorph is lean with a thin, delicate build and might have trouble gaining weight. A mesomorph is muscular with a hard, rectangular build and gains or loses weight easily. An endomorph is plump with a soft, round build and might have trouble losing weight. Most people do not fit perfectly into any one category. Although one type usually predominates, most of us are a combination of body types. Because everyone's body is unique, body typing and workout design are not exact sciences. However, knowing your predominant body type helps in developing an ideal exercise and diet plan to meet your goals. Each body type requires a different bodybuilding prescription. The regimen for an ectomorph differs from that for an endomorph because they are at opposite ends of the body type spectrum.

The *ectomorph* body type tends to have a fast metabolism and has a tough time gaining muscle mass. The prime goal of an ectomorph is weight gain, so his bodybuilding program must be prescribed with this in mind. Exercise should focus on mass-building workouts, using heavier weights and fewer repetitions. Calorie-burning cardio should be kept to a bare minimum. An ectomorph's diet should contain a surplus of calories from complex carbohydrate foods to encourage anabolic weight gain.

The *endomorph* is the exact opposite. This body type tends to have a slow metabolism that stores unwanted extra calories. The endomorph easily gains weight but struggles to lose body fat. The main goal for an endomorph is burning off excess body fat. For his purposes, exercise should include several cardio sessions per week. Weight training should be performed at a fast pace with a higher range of reps. Diet is critical for the endomorph. To promote fat loss, daily calorie intake must be less than the daily calorie expenditure. The diet should be high in protein and moderate in fat, with a moderate amount of complex carbohydrate foods. Snacking and empty calories should be avoided.

The *mesomorph* body type is genetically advantaged when it comes to building lean muscle mass. Often, the mesomorph looks like an athlete even without training. This body type can benefit from almost any training protocol. However, to realize maximum potential, the mesomorph must build on his genetically gifted foundation. The mesomorph thrives on challenge and variation. This body type responds well to an alternating exercise program, switching between a bulking-up phase to pack on mass and a cutting-up phase to define the added muscle.

If you need help in deciding your body type, you may utilize measurements such as body mass index, percent body fat, and resting metabolic rate.

Body mass index (BMI) is an indicator of total body fat based on height and weight that applies to adult men and women (see table 4.1). In simple terms, your BMI is calculated by dividing your weight (in kilograms) by your height (in meters squared). The BMI does have limitations, however, because it *overestimates* fat content in athletes and muscular persons.

Table 4.1 Body Mass Index

Less than 18.5	Underweight
18.5-24.9	Normal weight
25.0-29.9	Overweight
Above 30	Obese

A muscular person may have a BMI above 25 and would be categorized as being overweight according to table 4.1. Therefore, percent body fat (%BF) is a better indicator of fat content for bodybuilders. For example, a lean and muscular man standing 5 feet 11 inches (1.8 m) and weighing 200 pounds (91 kg) with 10 percent body fat has a BMI of 28 (i.e., overweight). He may be above average weight for his height, but with a body fat of 10 percent he is clearly *not* fat.

The simplest method of measuring body fat percentage is using a skinfold caliper. Follow the manufacturer's instructions, and record the skin thickness at three sites on your body (typically the upper arm, waist, and thigh). Calculate the average reading by adding all three measurements and then dividing by 3. The average body fat percentage for males is 15 percent, but a sleek six-pack of abs will show only if your body fat is below 10 percent. The skinfold caliper will give a rough estimate of your body fat, but this method lacks accuracy, and your calculation may be off by a few percentage points—not good if you're monitoring small changes.

Your local gym or doctor's office may offer more accurate assessments of BMI, percent body fat, and metabolic rate. Commonplace nowadays are airtight chambers that calculate body composition by measuring the volume of air a person's body displaces while inside the chamber. Other devices such as handheld calorimeters offer quick and accurate measurements of your resting metabolic rate. All you need to do is breathe into this device for several minutes while at rest, and, by measuring oxygen consumption, the device is able to calculate your metabolic rate. Measurements such as BMI, percent body fat, and metabolic rate are useful for determining your body type before starting your program as well as for monitoring the progress you make at regular intervals.

So, let's briefly discuss the three body-sculpting programs outlined in this book. If you're looking to pack on pounds of muscle fast, the mass generator program (chapter 7) is the plan for you. I have selected 14 of the best mass-building exercises and combined them into a three-day split-workout routine that hits the muscles hard while providing ample time for recovery and growth. To optimize muscle hypertrophy, you'll perform between 6 and 10 repetitions, using 70 to 80 percent of your one-rep maximum (1RM) weight on each exercise. The mass-generating diet will deliver a surplus of calories to give your muscles the fuel they need to grow.

If you're looking to lose unwanted body fat quickly, the body fat blitz program (chapter 10) is the plan for you. I have combined a selection of resistance and aerobic exercises into a four-day workout routine that increases your metabolic rate and melts away your fat stores. To maximize calorie use, you'll perform between 10 and 15 repetitions of each weight-training exercise, keeping the rest interval between sets under 60 seconds. The fat-loss diet aims to create a daily calorie deficit so that the negative caloric balance forces your body to burn fat stores to provide energy.

If you're looking to forge the ultimate physique, the hybrid hard body program (chapter 14) is the plan for you. This workout combines 30 of the most effective muscle-shaping exercises into a four-day split-training routine. I have included a couple of cardio sessions in the weekly schedule to tease off that fat layer and showcase your hard-earned muscle. The hard body diet provides enough nutrients to fuel muscle growth, while careful calorie control starves your fat stores. The hybrid system is a blend of techniques and a combination of bodybuilding styles that simultaneously stimulates muscle growth and promotes fat loss. In effect, with the hybrid system you get the best elements of the mass generator program (chapter 7) and the body fat blitz program (chapter 10), and then some.

SELECTING YOUR PROGRAM

When you begin a workout program, the first step is to choose a goal. Decide what you really want to change. If your main objective is to add some size to your guns or expand your chest measurement, then you should style your routine toward building mass. On the other hand, if your wish is to lose the spare tire around your waist and get a six-pack, then you should focus on burning calories. Can't decide? Come on, be honest with yourself! Jump on the scale, take a look in the mirror, and get out the tape measure. If you are overweight and your waist is bigger than your chest, I reckon you should be focusing on losing some lard rather than bulking up.

Table 4.2 Program Selection Algorithm

Body Type	Ectomorph	Endomorph	Mesomorph
BMI	<20	>30	20-30
Body fat	<10%	>15%	10-15%
Metabolism	Fast	Slow	Average
Gym experience	Low	Low	High
Goal	Gain mass	Lose fat	Advanced
Program	Mass generator	Body fat blitz	Hybrid hard body
After 6 months recheck BMI + %BF			

Several key objectives will guide you in selecting your personalized program. Also see table 4.2 for an algorithm for selecting which program is right for you.

> **Objective 1: Focus on your primary goal.** Your brain works best when it focuses on a single task. By choosing a specific target, you'll be slick and quick in cutting straight to the chase. To fine-tune your physique, identify exactly what your needs are. Do you want to gain muscle, torch body fat, or achieve both?

> **Objective 2: Coordinate exercise and diet.** Whether your quest is more muscle or less flab, you have two weapons at your disposal: exercise and diet. Exercise and diet are a tag team. They can function alone but work much better together. A low-calorie diet designed to shed body fat does not complement a mass-building exercise regimen. For best results, combine exercise and diet in the most effective way.

> **Objective 3: Tailor your exercise technique.** The exercise protocol for maximizing muscle growth is different from the protocol for slicing off body fat. By manipulating the ground rules and tweaking your technique, you can create a program that does exactly what you want it to do.

RECORDING YOUR DATA

I recommend you keep a journal documenting your progress. You will witness small measured changes before you'll see significant visual changes in the mirror. And documenting changes is an excellent source of motivation. You'll be recording data in two categories: shape and function. In the *shape* category, measure body weight using a scale; take body measurements—such as chest, arm, and thigh circumference—with a tape measure; and take a full-body photograph. Record your data at the beginning, then every four weeks as your body responds to the program. In the *function* category, measure muscle strength by recording the maximum weight you can lift for six repetitions during the last set of each exercise. The stronger the muscle becomes, the bigger it grows. To continue growing muscle, aim to increase the weight on each exercise by 5 percent every two weeks. You can document as much data as you like in your training journal, including daily food and water intake, workout time and duration, sleep schedule, body weight, body mass index, and percent body fat.

Plateau:
Any tips on how to break out
of a training plateau?

To make progress in bodybuilding, all the basic components—exercise, nutrition, rest, supplements, and so on—must fit together perfectly like the pieces of a jigsaw puzzle. If you're not witnessing positive changes in your physique, you'll need to carefully evaluate your workout regimen and dietary habits. For your exercise program, you should evaluate the amount of weight, the number of reps and sets, exercise selection, rest intervals, workout time, and recovery periods. For your nutrition program, you must consume the correct number of calories from the right food sources and partition the nutrients (protein, carbohydrate, fat) in the ideal proportions. If you are stuck in a training rut, the first thing you must identify is the exact goal that you're failing to realize: Is it strength, size, or fat loss? It's easier if you focus on fixing one fault at a time.

ADAPTING YOUR PROGRAM

Remember, *there is no single method to suit every individual body type.* Whichever program you select, it is just a basic blueprint. You need to adapt the framework to create a program that's specific to you on several levels. For instance, you'll calculate the amount or weight that *you* can safely lift for the appropriate number of repetitions on each exercise. You'll decide what days you work out and what time you train, depending on your work and domestic commitments. What's more, calculating your own personal nutrition plan is critical. Bear in mind that the calorie estimations provided are based on an average adult male with a sedentary, nonphysical job. However, individual calorie intake is dependent on several factors including age, occupation, sport, body type, and goals. The younger and more physically active you are, the higher your baseline daily calorie requirement. The older and less physically active you are, the lower your baseline daily calorie requirement. So your diet should be adjusted to a calorie intake that matches your activity level and metabolic rate. The daily calorie requirement will be higher if your job involves hard labor or if you are a teenager with a high metabolism.

UPGRADING YOUR PROGRAM

As your body changes, you need to upgrade your program by making adjustments to the basic blueprint. Every month when you record your measurements, you'll need to make the appropriate changes and adapt your program accordingly. For instance, as you get stronger, you'll need to lift heavier weights, and as your body weight changes, you'll need to adjust your calorie intake. Evolution is key to progress, and you should strive to evolve every month. If you do not upgrade the program, your body will not continue to change. It's important to monitor your progress. If you are not gaining muscle, eat more. If you are not losing body fat, eat fewer calories. To facilitate increasing muscle mass, I recommend increasing your daily calorie intake by 10 percent every month up to an additional 50 percent on top of your baseline intake. Upping your calorie intake dramatically will likely result in the excess calories being stored as fat, whereas a sequential, gradual increase in calorie intake feeds muscle growth. *Small, smart steps are best.*

MODIFYING YOUR PROGRAM

The programs in this book are designed with modification in mind. Every reader is a unique person. And I appreciate that. You are allowed to substitute and interchange exercises and meals from one program to another—provided the basic blueprint stays the same. If you don't like a particular exercise in your program, you can substitute another exercise that works the same muscle group. If you dislike the ingredients of a certain meal, you can select a different meal provided it provides the same nutritional content.

PROGRESSION

All three body-sculpting programs described in this book are interchangeable. As you make progress, you can shift from one program to another depending on your needs. For example, let's say you've shed all your unwanted body fat after six months on the body fat blitz program, and now you want to add muscle mass. All you need to do is slip seamlessly over to the mass generator program. Then after another six months when you've gained a solid foundation of muscle, you can progress to the hybrid hard body program. Make simple, sensible, and strategic steps.

———————————

The bodybuilding programs in this book describe in detail the workout regimens and nutrition plans necessary to build muscle and burn body fat. Each program serves its own purpose, and the programs are interchangeable depending on your needs. Your bodybuilding prescription must be individualized. Having read this chapter, you should now have a clear idea which program is best suited to your body type. If your main goal is to gain muscle mass, I recommend you proceed to part II. If you want to lose body fat, proceed to part III. Alternatively, if you're ready for a more advanced program, then proceed to part IV.

Maximizing Muscle Mass

In part II, you'll be equipped with the complete package to maximize muscle mass. The focused contraction technique (chapter 5)—unique to this book—is the ultimate muscle-building stimulus. Every rep and every set of every workout serve a specific purpose. Muscle growth requires an anabolic environment, a state that promotes tissue repair. In chapter 6, you'll learn 12 simple steps toward gaining an anabolic advantage and optimizing your body's testosterone level. More testosterone means more muscle and a supercharged sex drive. The mass generator program (chapter 7) is my personal prescription for packing on pounds of muscle fast. Each exercise is handpicked to induce a surge in size.

Mass Construction

The raw material you need to sculpt your body is muscle. Try this little experiment. Next time you walk past the meat counter at your butcher or supermarket, buy a pound (.5 kg) of ground beef. Now if you were to mold that raw material onto your biceps, then you'd realize that a pound of muscle is a lot of meat. Generating that extra muscle is no small feat, but it is easier if you employ the right strategy. For instance, you will add muscle mass more quickly when you work larger muscle groups, such as the legs, chest, and back. What's more, a muscle will grow more effectively if you stimulate all of its anatomic sections. In chapter one, you learned the five basic rules to lift by—namely the number of repetitions, amount of weight, number of sets, rest intervals, and workout duration. So let's develop these principles further and discuss my strategy for mass construction by selecting and combining the best bodybuilding exercises that stimulate muscle growth.

Focused contraction training (FCT) is an intelligent exercise system designed to generate the ultimate muscle-building stimulus. In FCT, every rep and every set of every workout serve a specific scientific purpose. Each exercise is handpicked to build and sculpt your body. FCT requires you to train with your brain by engaging your mind first and then your muscle.

Central to FCT is the focused contraction technique, which has two key strategies. The first is that your mind must be completely focused on the muscle you are working; the exercise demands your undivided attention. Think of your muscle as an electrical appliance—plug it in and turn it on. The second strategy is that your muscle must be contracting during every phase of the repetition. Keep the muscle being worked under tension, and don't let it relax at any time. Remember that it's time under tension that makes muscle grow. When you combine these two strategies, you get a focused contraction—the ultimate muscle-building formula.

The principles of FCT are as follows:

- Work one muscle at a time.
- Move one joint at a time.
- Use one limb at a time.
- Use a short, safe range of motion.

I'll explain how these principles work. The first three assist your ability to focus. The brain works best when it focuses on one task at a time. The more specific the task, the more attention the task receives from the brain. The ideal exercise to generate a focused contraction is one that works a single muscle by moving one joint of one limb—for example, the biceps flexing the elbow of one arm. When all other muscles and joints are taken out of the game, the mind–muscle link is enhanced, and you can focus all your effort on generating the maximum possible muscular contraction.

The fourth principle—use a short, safe range of motion—ensures a continuous muscular contraction throughout the phases of the repetition. To keep tension on the muscle during an exercise, restrict the movement to a short range of motion. To illustrate this point, let's consider the biceps curl. As the weight is lowered and the elbow straightens, tension is temporarily removed from the biceps. When tension is off the muscle, it cannot generate an effective contraction. To prevent the biceps from taking a relaxation break at the bottom of the lift, stop 5 to 10 degrees short of full extension to retain tension on the muscle. Go ahead and feel the consistency of your biceps muscle contraction when your elbow is straight. Now compare it to when your elbow is bent. The muscle contraction is much harder with your elbow bent, isn't it? Because the biceps is at a mechanical disadvantage when the elbow is fully straight, it is prevented from contracting effectively. The same thing happens when your arms approach lockout during pressing movements. The tension is removed from the chest and deltoid muscles when the load switches over to the triceps. If you want to keep tension on the chest during bench presses and on the deltoid during shoulder presses, pause the repetition just short of the full lockout position.

Another aspect of this fourth principle is that a short range of motion is also a safe range of motion. At the extremes of joint movement, your anatomy is pushed to the limit. Your muscles, tendons, and joints are most vulnerable at the extremes of limb movement. In these positions, there is a higher risk of damage, particularly when lifting a weight. So a short, safe range of motion serves two purposes: It helps maintain a continuous muscular contraction, and it minimizes the risk of injury.

The principles of FCT do not apply to all exercises. For example, FCT does not apply to the deadlift because it is a multijoint exercise that requires all four limbs and works numerous muscle groups. But if the FCT technique is incorporated into your workout, you will generate a focused muscle contraction. Before you apply these principles to individual exercises, you need to address a few questions: Which type of exercises should you choose? In what order should you perform the exercises? How many exercises are needed to shape each individual muscle?

Exercise vs. Diet: What's more important for building muscle, exercise or nutrition?

The answer is exercise! Exercise makes a muscle work, uses up its energy store, and causes microscopic damage to the muscle fibers. After exercise, the muscle needs nutrients to recover—that is, to restock energy stores and repair damage. During the recovery process, the muscle adapts by getting bigger and stronger. The stimulus for muscle adaptation is exercise. In other words, you cannot build muscle unless you work out. Even if you consume a boatload of supplements, your muscles will not grow without exercise.

EXERCISE TYPE

When you consider all the possible exercise variations—barbells, dumbbells, machines, cables, and so on—the list of choices is as fat as a small town's phone book, with more exercises than you'll ever need. The bottom line is there are two basic types of resistance exercise: isolation exercise and compound exercise.

As the name suggests, an isolation exercise isolates one muscle and typically involves motion at one joint. Examples include one-arm biceps curls, leg extensions, and shoulder raises. In contrast, a compound exercise requires the coordinated action of two or more muscle groups with motion occurring at more than one joint. Examples of this type of exercise include squats, bench presses, and shoulder presses.

By tradition, compound exercises are considered strength builders, and isolation exercises are favored for shaping muscles. To provide your muscles with the ideal stimulus, your exercise regimen should include both types of exercise.

Now let's look at the sequence you should use in your workout.

EXERCISE ORDER

The order in which you perform your exercises can make a huge difference. To achieve the best muscular contraction, you'll need to focus your mind entirely on the muscle being worked. When this occurs, the muscle sends a message of approval back to your brain. This signal from the muscle back to the brain enhances the forward link from mind to muscle. In other words, your brain senses that the muscle is working and, in turn, is able to generate a more focused contraction. This is called the mind–muscle feedback loop. When you generate this positive feedback, your muscle can work harder, which results in greater muscular growth. If you can't sense the muscle contracting, you have no way of knowing if you're actually making it work. If that's the case, you're wasting your time on that exercise.

To help generate the mind–muscle feedback loop, my exercise regimen prescribes an isolation exercise before a compound movement. I prefer to call the isolation movements primer exercises. The primer serves several purposes. First, it is a warm-up exercise to get the blood flowing through the muscle. Second, it makes it easy to develop the mind–muscle link right off the bat. Third, the muscle is primed and ready for the compound exercise. Finally, with the muscle already fatigued from the primer exercise, you don't need to lift as much weight during the compound exercise, which reduces the risk of injury associated with too heavy a weight.

When you group exercises for different body parts, remember to work from big to small. Train larger body parts such as the chest, quads, back, and shoulders before training smaller muscle groups such as the biceps, triceps, and calves. These smaller body parts function as support muscles for basic lifts such as bench presses, shoulder presses, rows, and squats. If you tire these smaller muscles first, they won't be able to assist effectively on the big exercises, which means the larger muscles won't get an adequate workout. Another benefit of training big to small is that the smaller muscle group will be warmed up and ready when its turn comes.

EXERCISE NUMBER

How many exercises does it take to shape each muscle group? The answer depends on the size of the muscle in question.

Small Muscles   Smaller (limb) muscles such as the biceps and triceps attach to bone through thin, cordlike tendons. Because their narrow tendons attach to a single point on the bone, the biceps and triceps generate motion in one plane only—bending and straightening the elbow. All you need to do to effectively work the biceps or triceps is to perform a single movement. Biceps curls and triceps presses will effectively build those muscles, whether you use a barbell, dumbbell, or machine.

Large Muscles   Larger (torso) muscles such as the deltoids, pectorals, and latissimus possess fanlike tendons that attach over a larger bony surface. These muscles are capable of generating movement in more than one direction. Thus, building these larger muscle groups requires a combination of exercises that work the muscle in several planes of motion.

To experience this type of fanlike tendon, examine the deltoid muscle of your shoulder. It's divided into three portions. In the front, the muscle attaches to your collarbone (clavicle). At the side, the lateral head attaches to the bone edge at the outer tip of your shoulder. Behind, the rear head attaches to your shoulder blade. Each part of the deltoid muscle serves its own function. The front deltoid raises your arm out in front of you. The lateral deltoid lifts your arm out to the side. The rear deltoid pulls your arm backward and behind. Feel each portion of the deltoid contract as you perform these three movements.

When a muscle has multiple sites of attachment, it's not possible to target all aspects of the muscle with a single exercise. To build all three sections of the deltoid muscle, you need to target each portion separately. Although the shoulder press might be considered the gold-standard shoulder exercise, it works only the front portion of the muscle. You have to incorporate a side lateral raise and a rear deltoid exercise for proportioned deltoid development.

Muscle Proportion   A proportionately developed muscle not only looks better but functions better too. Remember that the job of any muscle is to move a joint—the junction between two bones—and that each muscle that moves a given joint should be equally developed to optimize motion at that joint. It upsets the mechanics of a joint if one muscle is disproportionately stronger than its partner. Muscle balance is critical for proper joint function. For example, to optimize motion at the shoulder joint, all three heads of the deltoid muscle must be equally developed. This concept is of paramount importance when it comes to exercise selection.

The principle of muscle balance applies to all joints. Consider your elbow joint. Motion at this joint requires the coordinated action of the biceps muscle at the front and the triceps muscle behind. When the biceps muscle contracts, the elbow bends; when the triceps contracts, the elbow straightens. Each muscle causes motion in the opposite direction. When you bend the elbow, the biceps is called the agonist muscle, and the triceps is called the antagonist. When you straighten the elbow, the roles are reversed. Another example of agonist and antagonist muscles are the quadriceps and hamstring muscles that straighten and bend the knee joint.

If the agonist muscle is stronger or weaker than its antagonist, the muscles become imbalanced. This upsets joint mechanics and thus increases the chance of injury. When constructing your exercise regimen, be sure to select exercises that develop each muscle group equally and in proportion.

The concept of muscle balance and its relationship to optimizing function also applies to anterior–posterior muscle pairs in the torso core groups; for instance, the abdominals bend your torso forward, while the lumbar muscles extend the torso backward. Similarly, it is important to develop muscle balance and proportion between your upper body and lower body.

EXERCISE SELECTION

An effective bodybuilding program consists of a series of exercises that work all major muscle groups. For each individual muscle, there are only one or two basic movements. The chest muscles, for instance, can be worked with bench presses or chest flys. However, when you incorporate variation, the number of possible chest exercises becomes huge. Bench presses can be performed with the bench flat or tilted at an incline (head up) or a decline (head down) to work different areas of the pectoral muscle. The movement can be performed using a standard barbell, two dumbbells, or a machine. In other words, bench presses can be performed at three different angles using three different pieces of equipment. Do the math. The bench press has nine possible exercise variations. And that doesn't take into account the different types of machines, such as the Smith, Hammer, Nautilus, and so on.

Table 5.1 summarizes the different types of exercises for individual muscle groups. For variety, you have the choice (in most cases) of using free weights—barbell or dumbbells—or machines. The list includes exercises that I consider effective and safe when performed using the correct technique. I have excluded some exercises intentionally, either because I consider them biomechanically less effective or because they could do more harm than good. For example, upright rows and overhead triceps extensions place unnecessary stress on the shoulder joints. Dumbbell kickbacks will work the triceps, but there are better, more effective exercises to incorporate in your triceps workout. I have applied the same key principles of exercise efficacy and safety to all the exercise programs included in this book. I want you to get maximum results with minimum risk of injury.

Chest   Now, you should not be performing nine variations of bench presses during your chest workout. That would be overkill. It's also a waste of time to duplicate the exact same exercise because this provides no additional benefit. Apply the principles described earlier. First, select an isolation primer exercise, such as the chest fly, and a compound strength exercise, such as the bench press. Then select a variation of each exercise to target different areas of the chest muscle. For example, perform chest flys on a flat bench to work the midchest. Then perform the pressing movement with the bench at an incline of 30 to 45 degrees to target the upper portion of the chest. If you want to add a third exercise, add a decline movement to work the lower chest. Get the idea? Whether you perform each exercise with free weights (barbell or dumbbells) or on a machine is a matter of personal preference and availability of equipment. Ideally, you should use a combination of free weights and machine exercises.

The same principles apply when selecting exercises for the shoulders and back. Because there are several different parts to these large muscles, choose exercises that target different regions of the muscle group.

Table 5.1 Isolation and Compound Exercises for Specific Muscle Groups

Muscle group	Isolation exercises	Compound exercises
Chest	Chest flys using DB or machine; a flat bench targets the midchest, an incline bench targets the upper pecs, and a decline bench works the lower chest Cable crossovers	Bench presses using BB, DB, or machine; a flat bench works the midchest, an incline bench works the upper chest, and a decline bench hits the lower pecs
Shoulders	Deltoid raises using DB, machine, or cable; raise to the side for the lateral deltoid, to the rear for the posterior deltoid, and to the front for the anterior deltoid	Seated front shoulder presses using BB, DB, or machine Trapezius shrugs using BB, DB, or machine
Back	Lower back extensions, flat or inclined Pullovers using DB or machine	Cable pull-downs Chin-ups Rows using BB, DB, or machine
Abs	Sit-ups, flat or on a decline Floor crunches Cable or machine crunches Twisting sit-ups or crunches for the obliques	Leg raises performed hanging, on a decline, or using a machine
Quadriceps	Leg extensions (machine)	BB squats Machine squats (e.g., hack squats) Leg presses
Hamstrings	Seated or lying leg curls (machine) Standing leg curls (machine)	Straight-leg deadlifts using BB or DB
Calves	Seated (bent-knee) calf raises	Standing calf raises Donkey (straight-leg) calf raises
Biceps	Preacher curls using BB or DB Machine curls Concentration curls using DB or cable	Standing biceps curls using BB or DB Seated DB curls
Triceps	Cable triceps push-downs using bar or rope attachment Machine triceps push-downs	Close-grip BB bench presses Dips using parallel bars or machine
Forearms	Wrist curls using BB or DB Reverse wrist curls using BB or DB	Reverse-grip biceps curls using BB Hammer curls using DB

BB = barbell; DB = dumbbell

Shoulders For the shoulder, use isolation movements, such as lateral deltoid raises, to work the outer (side) portion of the deltoid, combined with compound movements, such as shoulder presses, to target the front portion of the deltoid muscle. If you wish to add a third shoulder exercise, select rear

Free Weights or Machines?

Free weights are considered the gold-standard gym equipment. And free weights are probably superior for sport-specific training where speed, power, and technique are paramount. However, when it comes to building and sculpting muscle, a weight is a weight. Your muscle doesn't know whether the weight source is a barbell, dumbbell, cable, or machine. Probably the best bodybuilding workout is one that combines free weights and machines. One drawback of certain machines is that friction between the moving parts prevents a smooth motion during the movement. But on the whole, machines can provide numerous benefits for bodybuilders.

1. User friendly: Machines are easier to use and technically less demanding.
2. Variety: Machines offer a wide choice of exercise variations.
3. Options: Machines offer different grip and stance options.
4. Convenience: Many machines let you avoid the hassle of loading and unloading weight plates.
5. Resistance: Machines and cables provide a fairly constant load that is unaffected by gravity.
6. Safety: Machines are safer, with a lower risk of injury.
7. Intensity: Many machines allow you to train to failure without the need for a spotter.
8. Targeting: Machines can target areas of the muscle that free weights cannot.

deltoid flys to work the posterior (rear) section of the muscle. You can target the trapezius muscle with the shrug exercise, using a barbell, dumbbells, or machine.

Back   For the back muscles, select an isolation exercise, such as extensions, for the lower back, then perform compound movements, such as chin-ups, pull-downs, or rows, to work the upper back muscles. By changing your grip, your hand spacing, or the angle of pull, you can target different regions of the upper back musculature. Wide-grip pull-downs or chin-ups work the outer latissimus flare. Rowing exercises tend to add thickness to the inner (central) portion of the latissimus muscle. Pulling the weight toward your abdomen during rows targets the lower lats, whereas pulling the weight high toward the chest works the upper lats, lower trapezius, and rhomboid muscles.

Abdomen   Your waist is made up of two muscle groups: the rectus abdominis in the front and the obliques on each side. Sit-ups and crunches are isolation exercises that target the upper abdomen, and leg raises are compound movements that work the lower abdominals. If you incorporate a twisting motion, you'll work the oblique muscles, too.

Selecting exercises for the limb muscles differs slightly from selecting exercises to work the muscles of the torso. The principles of isolation and compound exercises apply to the upper arm and thigh muscles, but the individual muscle groups are not subdivided into different target regions.

Legs   To work the quadriceps muscle at the front of the thigh, combine leg extensions (an isolation exercise) with a compound exercise, such as squats or leg presses. The hamstring muscles at the back of the thigh can be built effectively using leg curls, an isolation exercise. Add compound straight-leg deadlifts if required, but remember that the hamstrings are also worked during compound quadriceps exercises, such as squats and leg presses. When it comes to working the calf muscle, there are two basic types of calf raises. One is done with the knees straight (standing calf raises, donkey calf raises) and the other with the knees bent (seated calf raises). The difference in effect between the two positions is negligible when it comes to developing the calf muscles. However, in the seated position, no stress is placed on the lower back. And, because the knees are fixed, motion occurs exclusively through the ankle joint, which makes seated calf raises an isolation exercise.

Arms   Exercises for the biceps and triceps muscles of the upper arm also can be subdivided into isolation or compound movements. But because these muscles are smaller, they can be built effectively with one exercise each. I prefer isolation movements, such as preacher biceps curls and triceps push-downs, using a machine or cable equipment. It's important to remember that the biceps is worked during compound exercises that target the back and that the triceps is used in all pressing movements for the chest and shoulders. That's why I question the need for specific, additional compound exercises for the biceps and triceps.

If you wish to strengthen your forearm muscles, there are two forms of isolation exercise. Wrist curls (flexion) performed with a barbell or dumbbell work the front or inner part of the forearm. Reverse wrist curls (extension) build the back or outer muscles. Don't forget that the forearm muscles are worked whenever you grip a bar. Consequently, the forearms experience a compound-type exercise during most upper body workouts.

In this chapter we've focused on selecting and combining the best bodybuilding exercises that stimulate muscle growth. However, the biological process of muscle hypertrophy won't occur unless you provide the necessary anabolic ingredients. Just as a plant needs sunshine and water to grow, your body has a list of demands that must be met. In the next chapter, you'll learn 12 steps to optimize your body's anabolic environment.

Gaining an Anabolic Advantage

Anabolism is the process of tissue repair and growth. Your body must be in an anabolic state to build muscle. Intense exercise stimulates muscle growth, but that's only the spark that starts the anabolic process. The metamorphosis of muscle mass requires the right fuel intake, anabolic hormones, and time. The anabolic process is just like cooking a meal—you put together the ingredients, turn up the heat, and wait.

You can take advantage of the anabolic state—that magical place where muscle is made—by following these 12 steps:

1. Be protein positive.
2. Consume complex carbohydrate.
3. Count on calories.
4. Add water.
5. Recharge to get large.
6. Use the anabolic window.
7. Make use of supplements for size.
8. Keep away from cardio.
9. Turn up testosterone.
10. Switch on growth hormone.
11. Put insulin to work.
12. Work your body type.

In this chapter, we look at each of these steps in more detail and incorporate them into the ultimate mass-building program.

BE PROTEIN POSITIVE

Proteins are the building blocks of body construction. You can't build a house without adequate raw materials, and you can't build muscle without protein. The amino acid components of protein are the bricks your body uses to repair and build muscle after exercise. Protein is rich in nitrogen, so high protein intake ensures a positive nitrogen balance. If your body is holding more nitrogen than it's excreting, it's in that magical anabolic state, and you're on track to add muscle mass.

To get your fill of amino acids, aim for 1 to 1.5 grams of protein per pound (.5 kg) of body weight spread evenly over five or six meals per day. A 180-pound (82 kg) bodybuilder, for example, requires a minimum of 180 grams of protein a day, or 30 grams in each of six meals. Your intestinal tract is unable to absorb more than 50 grams of protein at once, so divide your daily intake over several meals. If you consume too much protein at one sitting, some of it won't be absorbed and will go to waste.

Foods high in protein include beef, poultry, fish, egg whites, milk, and whey. The easiest way to calculate your protein intake is to read the food label. As a rule of thumb, lean beef, chicken, turkey, and fish contain 6 to 7 grams of protein per ounce. A large egg white contains 6 grams of protein, and milk contains 1 gram of protein per fluid ounce.

Consuming enough protein at regular intervals throughout the day ensures an adequate supply of amino acids and provides a positive nitrogen balance. This creates an anabolic stimulus, which activates protein synthesis for muscle building and leads to faster recovery. And if you want to be big, you have to be anabolic!

CONSUME COMPLEX CARBOHYDRATE

If protein is the brick of body construction, carbohydrates are the cement. These complex sugar molecules stimulate the release of insulin, a potent anabolic hormone that drives amino acids into muscle cells, where they are used for repair. Once your daily requirement of protein is met, carbohydrates generate weight gain.

Carbohydrates are the body's preferred source of energy. After exercise, the body's storage tank of carbohydrates (muscle glycogen) depletes. When you eat plenty of carbohydrate, these energy tanks fill up and encourage the body to hold onto protein to build new muscle. If you skimp on carbohydrate, the tank empties quickly, forcing the body to burn protein for fuel instead of using it to repair muscle.

To add mass to your physique, you'll need to consume 1.5 to 2 grams of complex carbohydrate per pound (.5 kg) of body weight each day. A bodybuilder weighing 180 pounds (82 kg) requires at least 270 grams per day, or 45 grams in each of six meals.

Quality sources of complex carbohydrates include potatoes, rice, pasta, yams, oatmeal, whole-wheat bread, and vegetables. To provide your body with the best anabolic environment for gaining muscle mass, partition your daily food intake in the ratio of 50 percent carbohydrate, 40 percent protein, and 10 percent fat.

COUNT ON CALORIES

To gain muscle, you must be in a positive caloric balance. The way your body uses the protein you eat is directly related to your calories. When your calorie intake remains slightly higher than your daily energy requirement, protein is used to build muscle. If your calorie intake is consistently low, your body burns fat and protein for energy. This works fine for losing body fat, but it's not the way to add muscle mass.

A good way to keep your calorie level adequate is to calculate your maintenance daily calorie requirement (your body weight in pounds × 10, or your body weight in kilograms × 22), then add an extra 10 percent of that value. For example, if you weigh 200 pounds (91 kg), your estimated maintenance daily intake is 2,000 calories. An additional 10 percent (200 calories) brings your daily calorie total to 2,200 calories. Add the extra 200 calories by consuming 50 more grams of carbohydrate.

Monitor your progress using a scale. If your weight isn't moving up after a week or two, you don't have enough calories to grow. Increase your calorie intake by another 5 percent each week until your weight starts climbing in the right direction. The gradual 5 percent increase in calorie consumption is to ensure your weight gain comes from adding new muscle and not from laying down body fat.

ADD WATER

Muscle is 70 percent water, so maintaining your body's hydration ensures maximum muscle cell volume and helps muscular growth. Failing to drink enough water can adversely affect your gains in muscle mass. When the body dehydrates, water exits muscle cells, which sends the body into an antianabolic muscle-wasting state. A well-hydrated muscle is an anabolic muscle.

Begin hydrating your body first thing in the morning. Remember that an eight-hour overnight sleep is equivalent to one-third of a day, during which time you consume no fluids. Drink at least half a liter of water upon waking. Caffeine drinks such as coffee and tea have a diuretic effect, squeezing water out of the body, so if you enjoy a caffeine fix—and that's okay—be sure to restock your fluid balance.

Under average environmental conditions, the body needs a gallon (nearly 4 L) of water per day. In warmer climates, the daily water requirement increases to replace fluid lost through sweating. And although your work environment may be pleasantly cool during summer, air conditioning systems slowly dehydrate the body.

Keeping your body hydrated during exercise is essential. Water is all you need to replenish body fluids, provided your workout lasts less than an hour. Sports drinks containing added electrolytes, such as sodium and potassium, are more beneficial to athletes who exercise for longer periods without eating. As long as you're in and out of the gym within an hour, there's no real advantage in consuming these formulated drinks during your workout.

RECHARGE TO GET LARGE

You need downtime for muscle repair and recovery. You simply must get adequate rest if you want to grow. During exercise, muscle protein breaks down, and to restore protein balance, muscle protein synthesis is increased for at least 36 hours. Furthermore, to repair the muscle fiber disruption induced by a heavy weights session, the exhausted muscle requires five days of complete rest. Exercise-induced muscle growth is the ultimate result of the restoration of muscle protein balance and the repair of muscle tissue damage.

Rest days are a key component of any mass-building program. When your body is resting, it is building muscle tissue and restocking its energy stores. Without sufficient rest, your body remains in a catabolic state of negative protein balance and negative energy balance. If you deprive your body of the rest required for anabolism, your muscles won't gain size or strength. If you want to get large, you've got to recharge.

Another key requirement for anabolism is sleep. Do you know why babies sleep most of the time? Because they are growing. You need at least seven hours of sleep each night if you want to optimize levels of your body's two most potent anabolic hormones—testosterone and growth hormone.

The best way to ensure an adequate and restful night's sleep is to develop a regular sleeping pattern. Go to bed every night at the same time, preferably eight hours before you have to wake up the next morning. With a regular sleep routine, your body becomes accustomed to a restful sleeping pattern. If you can't ensure at least seven hours of sleep at night, try taking a 30- to 60-minute nap during the afternoon or early evening. Daytime napping is a good way to prevent chronic sleep deprivation.

USE THE ANABOLIC WINDOW

An anabolic window of opportunity opens immediately after you work out. Your body is drained of energy and in desperate need of refueling. After a workout, the body is a sponge for soaking up nutrients. This is a great opportunity to provide a quick burst of nutrients to jump-start the recuperation process.

A bout of heavy resistance exercise degrades muscle protein and depletes muscle glycogen. As part of the muscle's anabolic response to exercise, muscle protein synthesis and glycogen resynthesis begin immediately. The sooner you provide the necessary protein and carbohydrate building blocks, the quicker the muscle repairs the protein damage and restocks its glycogen energy store.

Research shows that if you consume protein and carbohydrate immediately after training, you can gain more muscle mass than if you wait an hour or two after the workout. To take advantage of that nutrition window of growth, you'll need quick-acting liquid nutrients rather than a solid meal that sits in your stomach for several hours. By the time a meal of solid food is digested, the anabolic window of opportunity has closed.

As mentioned in chapter 2, the best way to produce a potent anabolic effect is to drink a protein and carbohydrate supplement within 30 minutes of your workout. The best protein to use is whey (the quickest-acting bioavailable protein), which rapidly dissolves into amino acids, giving the body a quick fix of building blocks to expedite growth and recovery.

MAKE USE OF SUPPLEMENTS FOR SIZE

Nutritional supplements can be extremely helpful in your quest for muscle mass. In today's busy society, many people are at work or away from home at least eight hours a day. Under such circumstances, it's difficult to provide your muscles with a regular dose of quality nutrients in the right amounts. It's just not convenient to spend several hours in the kitchen each day preparing five or six muscle-building meals. Still, if you want those muscles to grow after all your hard work in the gym, you simply must meet their demands for fuel. And this is where quality nutritional supplements are useful.

The consumption of nutritional supplements after resistance exercise provides a hormonal environment that favors muscle anabolism. Some supplements provide extra nutrients to top off your dietary intake, whereas others are intended to stimulate muscle growth. Meal-replacement formulas are a convenient substitute for meals of solid food. Rather than resort to a fat-loaded meal of fast food, a high-protein and low-fat meal-replacement drink is a healthier and often cheaper alternative.

Protein is a key anabolic ingredient, but it's not easy to consume 1 to 1.5 grams of protein per pound of body weight each day from solid food, which often requires cooking. However, help is at hand in the form of quality supplements, such as whey protein. Low-carbohydrate protein supplements are available in powder forms, ready-to-drink bottles or cans, and tasty protein bars. With all the high-quality, convenient sources of protein out there today, it's easy to keep your protein tank full.

When sport supplements are scientifically compared, creatine comes out as the clear winner in terms of increasing muscle size and strength. This high-grade anabolic muscle fuel restocks energy stores, boosts muscle cell volume, switches on protein synthesis, and stimulates the release of growth hormone. When creatine is consumed with whey protein immediately after a workout, the muscle gains are superior to those obtained with either supplement taken alone. In other words, creatine and whey protein work as an anabolic tag team when used together after training.

The amino acid glutamine also has many benefits for those participating in intense exercise. Glutamine promotes muscle recovery, stimulates the synthesis of glycogen, and boosts immune function. Generally, a protein-rich diet should provide your body with a sufficient supply of glutamine. However, supplementing your diet with 5 to 10 mg a day provides extra insurance and prevents the muscle loss associated with glutamine deficiency.

KEEP AWAY FROM CARDIO

Exercise is a paradox of sorts. It is an insult to the body that triggers a stress response, inducing temporary catabolism. During this antianabolic state, body tissue breaks down. Although short bursts of hard-core training stimulate new muscle growth, exercising too long and too hard causes an increase in the stress hormones cortisol, glucagon, and catecholamine. These catabolic hormones trigger the burning of glycogen and amino acids and cause the breakdown of muscle tissue.

If you want to live in an anabolic state and grow muscle, your workouts must be heavy and short. After an hour, you've lost your power and are entering a state of catabolism. Do only what is necessary to stimulate muscle hypertrophy, then get out of the gym and start the growth process. Step away from the stair machine, trot past the treadmill, and bypass the bike.

Aerobic exercise is great for improving overall health and promoting fat loss. But if your goal is to pack on muscle mass, then don't overdo your cardio. You won't gain weight if you're burning more calories than you're taking in.

Too much cardio hinders the bulking-up phase. If you're accustomed to playing basketball for an hour or so every day, you might need to change your habits a bit if you want to bulk up. It's fine to enjoy a short run or swim on the days you're not at the gym, but take into account the additional calories you've used. When you're trying to gain muscle mass, you always want to consume a surplus of calories.

TURN UP TESTOSTERONE

Testosterone is what makes men men. This male hormone boosts sex drive and builds muscle mass; it can make a difference in bed and at the gym. Testosterone is made in the testes; an adult male produces about 7 mg of testosterone each day, or almost 50 mg a week. The average level of testosterone for men is 500 nanograms per deciliter (ng/dl), although levels vary from 300 to 1,000 ng/dl, depending on age.

Testosterone Boost:
How can I boost my testosterone?

Fact: The average male body loses one pound (.5 kg) of muscle and gains one pound of fat every year after age 35. Why? Healthy aging is accompanied by a progressive reduction in the production of anabolic hormones such as testosterone and growth hormone. Starting at age 30, the male body begins to shut down its production, and the decline continues in the order of 10 percent per decade. However, there are five simple tricks you can use to turn up testosterone naturally.

1. Lift weights: Short bouts of intense exercise boost hormone production.
2. Cut the cardio: Too much cardio causes testosterone to dip.
3. Adequate sleep: Get at least seven hours a night.
4. Eat more meat: Testosterone levels increase more with meat-based protein than with dairy.
5. Stay lean: Testosterone levels are optimized when body fat is below 15 percent but not too low.

Men in their late teens and 20s have the highest peaks in testosterone levels, which means this is the optimal age for testosterone's anabolic effect. This doesn't mean that men over the age of 30 are significantly disadvantaged. In most men, the decline in testosterone level with age is a slow process; a plentiful supply remains for decades.

Testosterone has powerful anabolic actions that build muscle and reduce body fat. Testosterone

• increases lean muscle mass and bone density and cuts down on body fat;

• ensures a positive nitrogen balance by stimulating protein synthesis and improving protein utilization;

• enhances carbohydrate energy stores and promotes fat burning; and

• stimulates red blood cell production, which expands blood volume and improves oxygen delivery throughout the body.

There are ways to enhance testosterone naturally. Production of the hormone is stimulated by short bouts of intense exercise and at least seven hours of sleep each night. Testosterone levels are optimized when protein intake is high (at least 1 gram per pound of body weight daily) and body fat is below 15 percent but not too low. Prohormone supplements containing steroid precursors such as androstenedione can also elevate testosterone. Herbs such as *tribulus* and *fenugreek* contain plant sterols called saponins that may stimulate the release of luteinizing hormone (LH), causing testosterone production. These measures—regular exercise, adequate sleep, high-protein diet, low body fat, prohormone and plant sterol supplementation—will *not* increase your testosterone level above the normal range. The increases are small. However, small increases may be all you need to make a difference.

SWITCH ON GROWTH HORMONE

Growth hormone (GH) is a substance made naturally in the pituitary gland (located at the base of the brain). It's an anabolic hormone that stimulates growth of bone, cartilage, and other tissues, such as muscle. In fact, GH appears to affect the growth of just about every organ and tissue in the body. It promotes protein synthesis, nitrogen balance, amino acid uptake, and fat loss. It also has an anti-insulin effect in that it raises blood sugar.

Under normal circumstances, there is a nighttime peak in GH release about two hours after the onset of sleep. GH release is stimulated by several factors, including exercise; sleep; low blood sugar; creatine supplementation; and the amino acids arginine, lysine, ornithine, and tryptophan. Obesity blunts GH release.

Healthy aging in men is accompanied by a progressive reduction in the daily production of GH and testosterone. The age-associated decline in anabolic hormones begins at around 25 to 30 years of age and contributes to increased fat accumulation and diminished energy, strength, and muscle mass. The good news is that you can minimize this age-related deterioration in your body by maximizing your anabolic drive using the strategies outlined in this chapter.

Heavy resistance exercise is a potent stimulus for increasing circulating anabolic hormones. You can also stimulate the release of GH by getting adequate sleep, keeping your body fat low, and avoiding sugar-loaded foods. Supplementing your diet with creatine and amino acids might be of additional benefit in boosting endogenous GH.

PUT INSULIN TO WORK

Two other important hormones involved in muscle growth and fat loss are insulin and glucagon. These hormones (produced in the pancreas) regulate carbohydrate and fat metabolism.

Insulin is released when blood sugar (glucose) levels rise after a meal of carbohydrate. The hormone transports glucose into cells where it's used for energy or stored as glycogen. Simple sugars with a high glycemic index are absorbed quickly into the bloodstream, causing a rapid release of insulin. This overproduction of insulin causes some of the carbohydrates to be deposited as fat instead of being stored as glycogen. Insulin is also involved in muscle growth because it transports amino acids into muscle cells. To facilitate this process, you need to consume carbohydrate. The key is eating the right kinds of complex carbohydrate in the right amounts.

Glucagon opposes the effect of insulin. Glucagon is released when blood sugar is low, typically several hours after a meal is eaten. In response to low blood sugar levels, glucagon converts stored glycogen into glucose. Because the body is running low on carbohydrates, glucagon also signals the body to start burning fat for energy. The ratio of insulin to glycogen in your body determines whether you'll gain or lose weight.

You can control this ratio by adjusting the relative proportions of protein and carbohydrate in your diet. Partition your food in a way to burn fat and build muscle. To gain muscular weight, you'll need a higher ratio of insulin. Thus, your daily nutrient intake should contain a higher proportion of carbohydrate than it does protein. Ensure that your nutrient ratio is about 50 percent carbohydrate, 40 percent protein, and 10 percent fat. Each meal should contain 30 to 40 grams of protein and 50 to 60 grams of carbohydrate, depending on your daily calorie allowance. Remember that once you've met your daily protein requirement—at least 1 gram of protein per pound of body weight—it's the extra carbohydrate load that packs on additional mass.

If you wish to lose body fat, you'll need a lower ratio of insulin. To increase glucagon and decrease insulin, eat slightly less carbohydrate and more protein. A simple rule of thumb is to adjust your protein-to-carbohydrate ratio to between 1 to 1 and 1.5 to 1. Partition your food so that the nutrient ratio is 50 to 60 percent protein, 30 to 40 percent carbohydrate, and 10 percent fat. One problem with reducing intake of carbohydrate is the decline in energy level, but minor adjustments on a day-to-day basis will tell you what works best in your case.

Don't take nutrient partitioning to extremes by going on a zero carbohydrate diet in an attempt to lose more body fat. Under extreme low-carbohydrate conditions, muscular growth is virtually impossible because insulin levels are too low to transport amino acids into muscle cells. What's more, the body begins to break down its own protein—eating away at your muscles—in a desperate attempt to generate glucose for energy.

WORK YOUR BODY TYPE

Scientifically speaking, some factors that determine weight gain are *not* under your control, specifically age, ethnic origin, genetics, and body type. The basic blueprint for your body's outward appearance is determined by your genes—the information contained in your body's cells—and this genetic code cannot be altered. The components you can control, namely exercise and nutrition, must be utilized in a specific way if you want to add muscle mass.

The key to creating your own workout and nutrition program lies in understanding your body type and building a regimen that accommodates your unique form rather than trying to change it. If you customize exercise and diet to your specific body type, you'll achieve a more effective transformation.

As discussed in chapter 4, the three basic body types are ectomorph, mesomorph, and endomorph. An ectomorph, the type of body that would most benefit by gaining an anabolic advantage, is lean with a thin, delicate build. A person with this body type tends to have a fast metabolism and has a tough time gaining muscle mass—in other words, the typical hard-gainer. The prime goal of an ectomorph is weight gain, so the bodybuilding program outlined in this chapter has been prescribed with this in mind. If you are struggling to put on muscle, you need to address the important variables in your workout and dietary programs. For instance, your training sessions should be brief and heavy, with an emphasis on compound multijoint movements such as squats, bench presses, and chin-ups. One thing that novice trainers tend to forget is that you are more likely to gain mass if you build the large muscles such as the thighs, back, and chest. Dancing around the gym training biceps for an hour is unlikely to influence your body weight. Calorie-burning cardio should be kept to a minimum. In addition, your diet should contain abundant sources of quality protein and complex carbohydrate to ensure a surplus of calories to encourage anabolic weight gain. What's more, you must allow adequate rest for muscle recovery and growth. In short, to be anabolic you must lift heavy, eat well, and sleep a lot.

Now that you know how to heat up your anabolic furnace, you're ready to generate some serious muscle mass. In the next chapter we unveil your personal prescription for packing on pounds of muscle. Read on to discover an ultimate mass-generating workout and an advanced anabolic diet that induces dramatic surges in muscle size.

Mass Generator Program

In the preceding chapters, we look at the science behind building muscle, explain the importance of exercise selection, and itemize the ingredients necessary for anabolic muscle growth. Now it's time to put these mass-building theories into practice.

If you're looking to pack on pounds of muscle fast, this is the plan for you. I have selected 14 of the best mass-building exercises and combined them into a three-day split-workout routine that hits the muscles hard while providing ample time for recovery and growth. To optimize muscle hypertrophy, you'll perform between 6 and 10 repetitions, using 70 to 80 percent of your one-rep maximum (1RM) weight on each exercise. The mass-generating diet will deliver a surplus of calories to give your muscles the fuel they need to grow. You can expect to make significant muscular gains using this program; be sure to monitor and record your progress at regular intervals.

PROGRAM OVERVIEW

As the name suggests, the mass generator program is designed to build muscle mass. To maximize muscle hypertrophy, the program emphasizes heavier weights and lower reps. Perform three sets of each exercise, using weights equal to 70, 75, and 80 percent of your 1RM. After an initial warm-up set of 10 reps, increase the weight on the second set so that your muscles fatigue after 8 reps. For the final set, add more weight and squeeze out 6 reps to failure. To make your muscles work hard, keep rest intervals as short as you can. Take 60 seconds of rest between the first two sets and 90 seconds before the final heavy set.

As you gain experience with this program, you can make the workout harder and even more effective by incorporating the high-intensity techniques described in chapter 11. Always take necessary safety precautions. To avoid accidents, use a spotter when lifting to complete muscular failure, especially when using free weights.

Workout Plan

The mass generator workout routine uses a push–pull three-way split-training system. I'll explain how it works. Session 1 involves upper body exercises (chest, shoulders, triceps) that require you to *push*. Session 2 is a leg workout that targets your quadriceps, hamstrings, and calf muscles. Session 3 involves upper body exercises (back, biceps) that require you to *pull*. This sequence groups together body parts that share similar exercise biomechanics. For example, in session 1, the *push* exercises for the chest also recruit the deltoid and triceps muscles. So, in effect, working the larger muscle group serves as a warm-up for working the smaller muscle groups, which follows later in the same workout. Similarly, in session 3, the *pull* exercises for the back muscles recruit and warm up the biceps. Thus, the smaller muscle is already pumped and ready for action when its turn comes. The leg muscles have session 2 all to themselves, working the largest muscle group (quadriceps) first in the sequence. The upper abdominals are worked with session 1 and the lower abs during session 3.

Frequency

In this program, each muscle is exercised once every seven days. As you'll recall from chapter 1, your muscles need five to seven days to fully recover from an intense weightlifting workout. Space the three workout sessions evenly during the week (e.g., Monday, Wednesday, Friday). Perform your leg workout between the two upper body workouts; this allows more recovery time for those muscles that assist in both upper body sessions. Larger muscles such as the chest, shoulders, back, and quads are each assigned two exercises. Each exercise intentionally hits the muscle from a different angle. As a rule, an isolation exercise is used first, followed by a compound movement. Smaller muscles such as the biceps, triceps, and calves are assigned one exercise each.

Three workouts per week might not sound like much exercise. However, during each 40-minute workout, you're required to work *hard*. If you want to build mass, you must push yourself. By the third set on each exercise, you should be lifting the heaviest possible weight for six reps to failure using flawless form. Then, with less than two minutes of rest, you're beginning the first set of the next exercise. Trust me, if you're putting all your effort into this mass-building routine, you won't want to work out more than three days a week! You'll soon realize that the four rest days per week provided during this program are an absolute requirement. Muscle grows when it's resting; recharge if you want to get large.

There's no calorie-burning cardio in the mass generator program. Your muscles will grow bigger and faster if you rest them completely between workouts. Thus, aerobic exercise is optional during your mass-building program. If you want to do some low-intensity cardiorespiratory exercise on the days you're not lifting weights, that's fine. But if you end up burning more calories than you're consuming, you won't gain muscular weight.

Nutrition Plan

To gain mass, you need to consume more calories than you burn. Those extra calories fuel muscle growth. So, how many calories should you consume each day during your mass-building program? Well, the first thing to do is calculate your maintenance daily calorie requirement (body weight in pounds × 10, or your body weight in kilograms × 22), as listed in chapter 2. Then add an additional 10 percent to this amount to increase your daily calorie intake for mass-building purposes. This gives your body 10 percent more calories than it needs for energy production. The surplus calories are used to build muscle. As you make progress over time, your calorie requirement is likely to increase sequentially with your gains in muscle mass.

The 2,000-calorie sample meal plan in table 7.1 is a rough guide for someone who weighs 180 pounds (82 kg). The daily calorie intake is equivalent to an 1,800-calorie maintenance value (180 pounds × 10) plus 10 percent, which brings the calorie total to 1,980 calories.

The next step is fun—you get to decide what food sources your calories come from. To promote muscular gains, the nutrient ratio of your diet should favor carbohydrate. I recommend partitioning your intake as follows: 50 percent carbohydrate, 40 percent protein, and 10 percent fat. Once you've met your daily protein requirement for muscle growth (1 gram of protein per pound of body weight per day), it's the extra carbohydrate that adds muscle mass.

Table 7.1 Mass Generator Sample Meal Plan

Breakfast	Egg-white scramble: Mix five egg whites and half a yolk with 1 tbsp of nonfat milk. Cook in a nonstick pan coated with nonfat cooking spray. Serve on two pieces of whole-wheat toast. Drink one cup of black coffee or water.
	Calories: 350
Midmorning snack	Meal-replacement drink: Mix one sachet of a meal-replacement powder with 12 oz (360 ml) cold water in a blender.
	Calories: 340
Lunch	Beef meal: Cook 6 oz (175 g) of lean ground beef in a nonstick pan. Drain excess fat and water. Mix with steamed chopped carrots. Serve with a portion of pasta cooked in water and sprinkled with lemon juice and herbs. Drink a glass of ice water.
	Calories: 440
Midafternoon snack	Protein drink: Mix one serving of protein powder with 4 oz (120 ml) water and 4 oz nonfat milk. Add one whole banana. Blend at high speed for 30 seconds.
	Calories: 240
Dinner	Chicken meal: Prepare a skinless chicken breast by squeezing lemon juice over it. Grill until cooked. Serve with a portion of steamed brown rice and broccoli. 1 tbsp of tomato ketchup is optional.
	Calories: 380
Late-evening snack	One serving of low-fat cereal or granola with 6 oz (180 ml) of skim milk
	Calories: 250
Daily values (approximate)	Protein: 200 g (800 cal), 40%
	Carbohydrate: 250 g (1,000 cal), 50%
	Fat: 22 g (200 cal), 10%
	Total calories: 2,000

Progression is essential. Increase your calorie intake by 10 percent each month, up to a maximum of 50 percent above your daily maintenance requirement. The *gradual* increase avoids an excessive calorie load that could lead to gaining fat instead of muscle.

Adjusting the sample meal plan to your weight is easy. Remember that 1 gram of protein is 4 calories, 1 gram of carbohydrate is 4 calories, and 1 gram of fat is 9 calories. Keeping the nutrient ratio at 40 percent protein and 50 percent carbohydrate, 100 calories equals 10 grams of protein (40 calories) plus 15 grams of carbohydrate (60 calories). To increase or decrease the calorie content to match your body weight, add or subtract these amounts from the sample meal plan.

Adjust your protein intake by changing the amount of protein powder added to your midafternoon snack or by changing the number of egg whites at breakfast (one egg white contains 6 grams of protein). Similarly, by adjusting the portions of pasta or rice at lunch and dinner, you can increase or decrease your intake of carbohydrate. But remember that the nutrition values in the sample meal plan are only approximate. Always check nutrition labels on the products you eat because values vary among brands. Supplementing your diet with creatine (chapter 13) will also help your mass-building efforts.

Adjust the content of the sample meal plan to match your individual body weight, using table 7.2.

Table 7.2 Daily Calorie Intake Based on Body Weight (Mass Generator)

Body weight (lb)	Body weight (kg)	Calories per day	Protein	Carbohydrate	Fat
220	100	2,400	240 g (960 cal)	300 g (1,200 cal)	26 g (240 cal)
200	91	2,200	220 g (880 cal)	275 g (1,100 cal)	24 g (220 cal)
180	82	2,000	200 g (800 cal)	250 g (1,000 cal)	22 g (200 cal)
160	73	1,800	180 g (720 cal)	225 g (900 cal)	20 g (180 cal)
140	64	1,600	160 g (640 cal)	200 g (800 cal)	18 g (160 cal)

Nutrient ratio: 40% protein, 50% carbohydrate, 10% fat
Calorie values: 1 g protein = 4 calories; 1 g carbohydrate = 4 calories; 1 g fat = 9 calories
Daily calorie intake = (body weight in pounds × 10) + 10% *or* (body weight in kg × 22) + 10%

Progress Measurements

You'll be recording data in two categories: shape and function. In the first category, measure body weight using a scale; take body measurements—such as chest, arm, and thigh circumference—with a tape measure. In the second category, measure muscle strength by recording the maximum weight you can lift for six repetitions during the last set of each exercise. The stronger the muscle becomes, the bigger it grows. To continue growing, aim to increase the weight on each exercise by 5 percent every two weeks.

Hard-Gainer:
I just don't gain weight!

Some factors that determine weight gain, such as age, genetics, ethnic origin, and body type, are *not* under your control. You can control exercise and nutrition, and these two components must be utilized in a specific way in order to build muscle. If what you're doing is not working, then you need to rethink your game plan. With your nutrition program, gaining weight means consuming more calories. For most people, this is relatively easy: Eat as much and as often as you can. When it comes to your exercise program, approach it like a scientific experiment, and evaluate all the ingredients: the amount of weight, the number of reps and sets, exercise selection, rest intervals, workout time, recovery periods, and so on. One thing that novice trainers tend to forget is that you are more likely to gain mass if you build the large muscles such as the thighs, back, and chest. Dancing around the gym training biceps for an hour is unlikely to influence your body weight. Here are some simple training suggestions to boost muscle mass.

1. Stick with three or four workouts per week.
2. Complete your workout in under an hour.
3. Pick power exercises such as squats, bench presses, and deadlifts.
4. Lift as heavy as you can.
5. Stay away from cardio.
6. Do not overtrain.

Results

After six weeks on this program, you should gain four to six pounds (1.8-2.7 kg) of muscle mass—as much as one pound (.5 kg) per week. Now this might not sound like a lot of muscle, but try taking a pound of ground beef and forming it in the shape of a pectoral muscle—you'll see that a pound of meat *is* substantial. Now imagine spreading six pounds of beef all over your body. That's a serious gain in muscular size. After six weeks on this mass program, you'll add an inch (2.5 cm) to your chest circumference and a half-inch (1.25 cm) to your arm and leg measurements. What's more, this extra muscle should boost your strength by 10 to 15 percent on every exercise. As you gain size and strength, your calorie requirement will increase, so don't forget to adjust your diet plan accordingly.

So, enough talk already. Let's look at exercise techniques that forge a massive physique.

MASS GENERATOR EXERCISE PROGRAM

Routine: Push–pull three-way split
Cycle: Three days per week
Schedule: Monday, Wednesday, Friday
Goal: Increase muscle mass
Detail: 3 sets of 10, 8, 6 reps
Rest interval: 60 to 90 sec
Workout time: 40 min

Push Monday	
Chest	Dumbbell chest fly
	Incline bench press
Shoulders	Dumbbell lateral raise
	Barbell shoulder press
Triceps	Close-grip bench press
Abs	Decline sit-up

Legs Wednesday	
Quadriceps	Leg extension
	Barbell squat
Hamstrings	Leg curl
Calves	Standing calf raise

Pull Friday	
Back	Chin-up
	Barbell row
Biceps	Barbell curl
Abs	Incline leg raise

Dumbbell Chest Fly

Grab two dumbbells of equal weight and sit at the edge of a flat exercise bench. Lie back, keeping the dumbbells close to your chest. Stabilize your body by placing your feet flat on the floor. Push the dumbbells up into the start position with your palms turned toward each other (figure 7.1*a*). Begin the repetition by lowering the dumbbells out to the sides (figure 7.1*b*), bending your elbows slightly as the weights descend. Inhale as you lower the weight, and feel your chest muscles stretch. Stop when your elbows reach bench level. Hold the weight for one second in the bottom position, then squeeze the dumbbells back up and together, exhaling as you lift. Keep your elbows slightly bent and your palms turned toward each other. Move the dumbbells in an arc, as if you're giving someone a bear hug. To keep the tension on the muscles, do not touch the dumbbells together at the top.

> ▶ **CHECK IT!** Don't let your arms go below the level of the bench, as this places unwanted stress on your shoulder joints.

Chest flys can also be performed using machines with either a hand grip or elbow pads (chapter 14). Read the instructions printed on the machine for additional guidance.

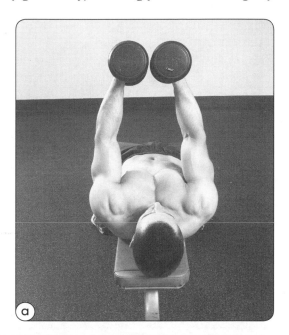

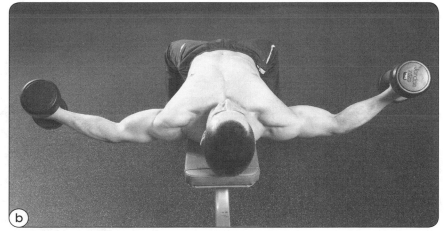

Figure 7.1 Dumbbell chest fly: *(a)* Hold dumbbells over your chest; *(b)* lower dumbbells to your sides.

Incline Bench Press

Lie back on an exercise bench tilted at an angle of 30 to 45 degrees (head up). Position your feet firmly on the floor. Take an overhand grip on the barbell with palms turned forward. Your hands should be slightly wider than shoulder-width apart. With your elbows locked straight, hold the bar in the start position above your chest (figure 7.2*a*). Begin the repetition by bending your elbows. Lower the weight slowly to the midpoint of your chest, just above the nipple line (figure 7.2*b*). Inhale as you lower the weight. Let the bar touch your chest, and hold it for one second. Do not let the bar rest on your chest. Without bouncing the barbell, push the weight vertically upward to the start position. Hold the bar with your elbows straight for one second. Repeat.

▶ **CHECK IT!** Remember that the bar travels *vertically* up and down perpendicular to the *floor*, not your body.

You can also do this exercise using a Smith machine.

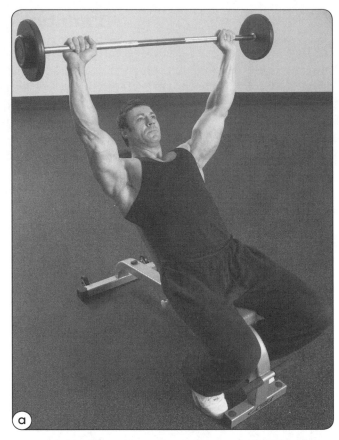

(a)

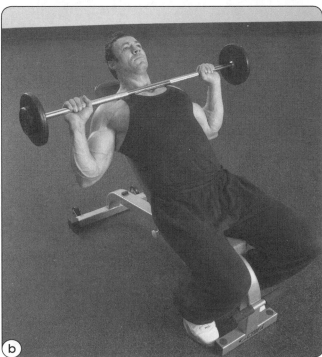

(b)

Figure 7.2 Incline bench press: *(a)* Hold the barbell over your chest; *(b)* lower the weight until the bar touches your chest.

Dumbbell Lateral Raise

Grab two dumbbells and stand upright with your feet about shoulder-width apart. Hold the dumbbells at arms' length just in front of your hips with palms turned toward each other (figure 7.3*a*). Raise your arms to your sides until they're level with your chin (figure 7.3*b*). Keep your palms turned down and your elbows slightly bent during the lift. Your arms should move directly out to the sides until your elbows are level with your shoulders. Hold that position for one second, then lower the weight slowly back to the start position. Keep your torso upright during the movement. A slight forward tilt is acceptable, but don't lean backward. You can also do this exercise while seated using dumbbells (chapter 10) or with one arm at a time using a cable attached to a low pulley (chapter 14).

▶ **CHECK IT!** Do not raise the dumbbells too high because this places undue stress on the shoulder joints. Your hands should be level with your chin, your elbows at shoulder height.

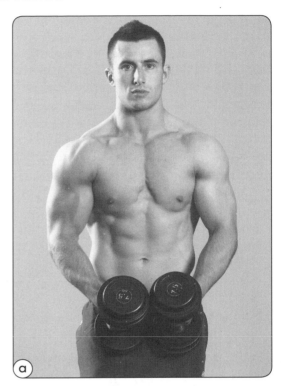

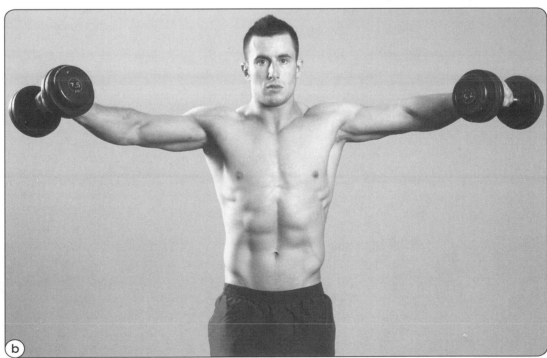

Figure 7.3 Dumbbell lateral raise: *(a)* Hold dumbbells in front of hips; *(b)* lift weights to the sides.

SHOULDERS

Barbell Shoulder Press

Sit on a bench with the backrest upright at a vertical angle. If the backrest is adjustable, tilt it back about 20 degrees to optimize body position. Firmly position your feet on the floor, and lean back onto the bench. Take a shoulder-width grip on the barbell with palms turned forward. Remove the barbell from the rack; position it overhead with elbows locked (figure 7.4a). From the start position, lower the weight slowly in front of your face until it touches your collarbone (figure 7.4b). Pause for one second, but don't allow the bar to rest on your upper chest. Push the bar vertically up until your arms are fully extended overhead. Pause for one second and then repeat.

▶ **CHECK IT!** Avoid behind-the-neck shoulder presses because they risk injury to your shoulder joints. Keep your hands in front where you can see them. Do not allow the weight to stray back and forth during the movement.

You can perform this exercise using dumbbells with palms turned forward, or using a seated front press machine.

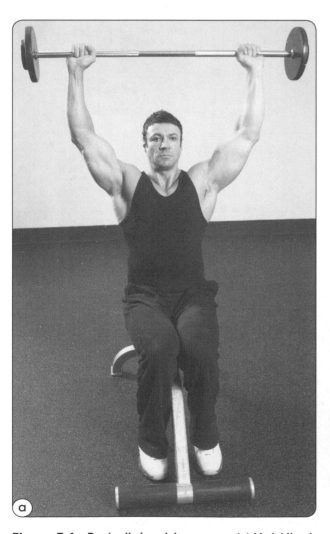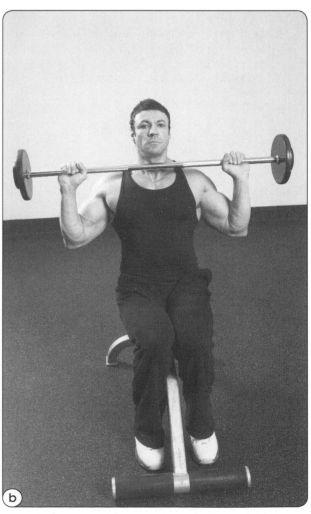

Figure 7.4 Barbell shoulder press: (a) Hold the barbell overhead; (b) lower the weight to your chest.

Close-Grip Bench Press

Lie supine on a flat bench; grab the barbell with an overhand grip, hands about four to six inches (10-15 cm) apart. In the start position, hold the barbell fully extended over your chest (figure 7.5*a*). Lower the barbell slowly in a vertical plane, bringing it close to your lower chest (figure 7.5*b*). Keep your elbows close to your sides as you lower the weight. Pause momentarily at the bottom, then press the bar upward until your elbows are fully extended. Squeeze the triceps for a count of one, then repeat.

▶ **CHECK IT!** Keep your buttocks in contact with the bench throughout the movement.

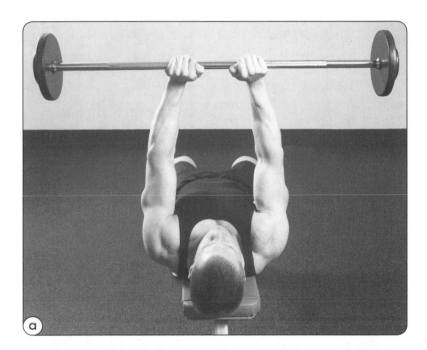

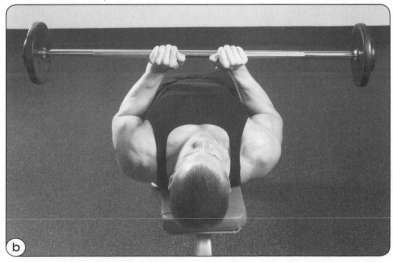

Figure 7.5 Close-grip bench press: *(a)* Hold the barbell over your chest; *(b)* lower the weight until the bar almost touches your chest.

Decline Sit-Up

Adjust a decline bench to a 20-degree angle in relation to the floor (head down). Hook your feet under the roller pad, and rest the back of your legs on the knee pad. Initially, sit upright on the bench so that your torso is upright and perpendicular to the floor (figure 7.6). You can hold your hands together behind your lower back or interlock them behind your head. Begin the exercise by lowering your torso slowly backward while contracting your abs. Lean back until your torso is almost parallel to the floor. Holding the bottom position, flex those abdominal muscles for one second. Crunch back to the start position, bending at the waist. In the top position, your body should be perpendicular to the floor, not touching your thighs. Hold in the contracted position for one count, then repeat.

▶ **CHECK IT!** Do not lean back too far. When tension is released from the abs, stress is placed on the lower back.

This is a great exercise for the upper and middle abdominal muscles. As you gain strength, you can increase the number of reps, tilt the bench at a steeper angle, or hold a small weight plate on your chest.

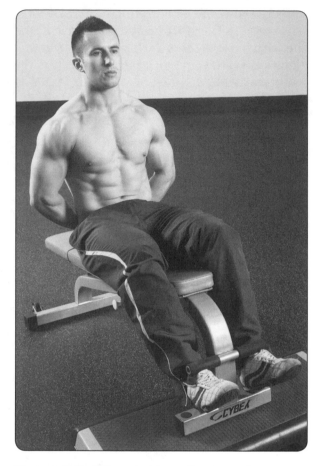

Figure 7.6 Sit upright on the bench.

Leg Extension

Sit at a leg extension machine. Adjust the backrest so that the backs of your knees fit snugly against the seat and your thighs are supported. Position your ankles under the roller pad. If the pad is adjustable, position it so it rests just above your ankles on the lowest part of your shins (figure 7.7a). Grip the handles on the machine for support. From the start position, contract your quadriceps to straighten your knees (figure 7.7b). Lift the weight all the way up until your knees are straight. Pause for one second at the top, making sure to flex your quadriceps. Lower the weight slowly until your knees are bent 90 degrees. Hold the weight momentarily in the bottom position, then repeat.

▶ **CHECK IT!** Do not let your hips rise off the seat. Avoid bending your knees beyond 90 degrees, as this will cause stress on the knee joint.

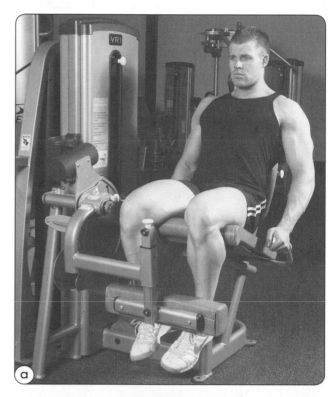

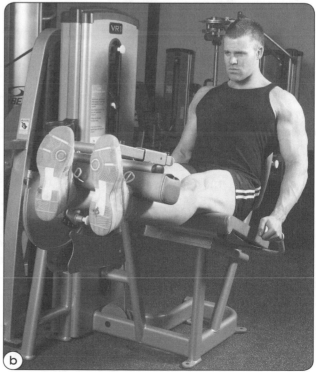

Figure 7.7 Leg extension: (a) Sit in leg extension machine; (b) straighten legs.

Barbell Squat

Position an empty barbell onto the squat rack, level with your upper chest. Load equal weight plates on either side of the bar, and secure them with safety collars. Note the center of the bar, and grip the bar in an evenly spaced overhand grip, hands wider than shoulder-width apart. Step under the bar, and position it comfortably on the upper portion of your back. Lift the bar off the rack, and carefully take one step away from the rack. Position your feet in line with your hips, and point your toes slightly outward. This is the start position (figure 7.8a). Begin the repetition by bending your knees and slowly lowering your hips straight down until your thighs are parallel to the floor (figure 7.8b). During the movement, be sure to keep your back straight, your chin up, and your grip firm to stabilize the bar on your shoulders. Don't lean too far forward because this places more stress on your lower back, and you might lose your balance. Once you reach the bottom position, push the weight up using your thighs and hips until your knees are straight. Inhale deeply during the descent, and exhale on the way up.

If you have trouble balancing during this exercise, place a one-inch (2.5 cm) thick wooden block under your heels. The squat is a great leg exercise, but it's also very demanding, requiring your full attention. Errors in technique can cause injury to your lower back or knees.

> **CHECK IT!** Avoid squatting below parallel position, as this can damage your knees.

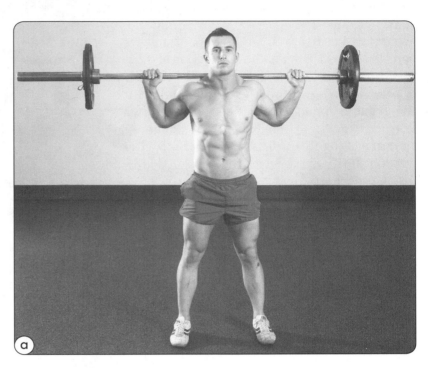

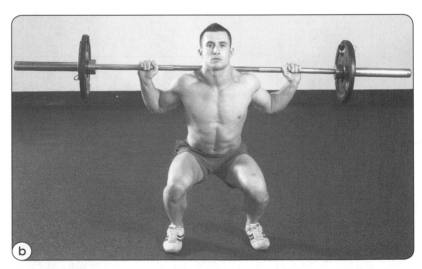

Figure 7.8 Barbell squat: *(a)* Stand with the bar across your shoulders; *(b)* lower your body until your thighs are parallel to the floor.

Leg Curl

Position yourself on a leg curl machine and rest the back of your ankles on the roller pads (figure 7.9*a*). Grip the handles for support. From the start position, curl the weight by bending your knees (figure 7.9*b*). Bring your heels toward your buttocks. Hold the contracted position for one second. Slowly lower the weight back to the start position so that your legs are almost straight. Hold momentarily and then repeat.

▶ **CHECK IT!** Do not lift your hips off the machine.

You can also do this exercise using a lying leg curl machine.

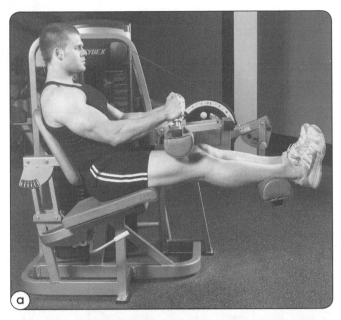

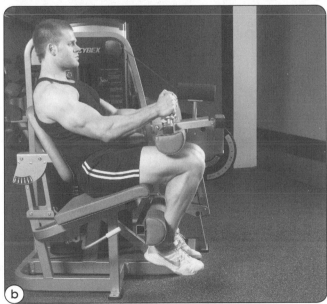

Figure 7.9 Seated leg curl: *(a)* Sit on a leg curl machine; *(b)* bring heels toward buttocks.

Standing Calf Raise

Position your shoulders under the bar of a Smith machine, and stand upright with your knees straight. Place the balls of your feet on the platform. Your feet should be directly beneath your hips. Slowly lower your heels as far as possible, stretching your calf muscles (figure 7.10a). Keep your back straight, and don't bend your knees. Hold the stretch in the lower position for one second. Lift the weight by raising your heels as high as you can (figure 7.10b). At the top position, contract your calf muscles hard and hold for one count (figure 7.10c). Lower the weight down slowly and then repeat. Variations of straight-leg calf raises are described in chapters 10 and 14.

▶ **CHECK IT!** Do not let your back hunch; keep your knees straight.

You can also perform this exercise using a standing calf raise machine.

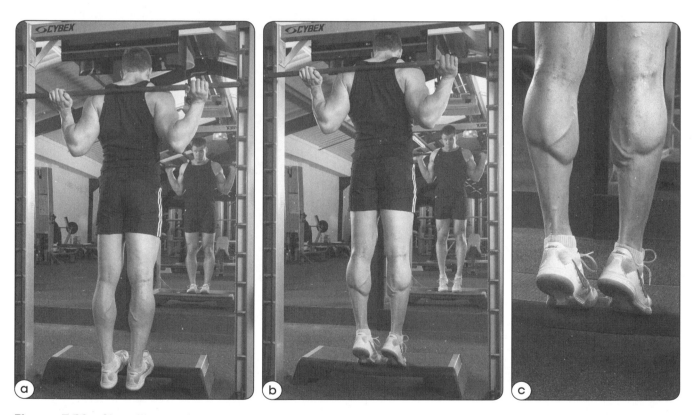

Figure 7.10 Standing calf raise: *(a)* Lower your heels; *(b)* lift the weight by raising your heels as high as possible; *(c)* contract calf muscles for one count.

Chin-Up

Grasp an overhead bar with an overhand grip, hands slightly wider than shoulder-width apart. Hang at arms' length, then lift your feet off the floor so that your body weight is suspended from your arms (figure 7.11a). Bend your knees slightly and lock one foot over the other, behind the plane of your body. From the start position, pull your body slowly upward until your chin touches the bar (figure 7.11b). Think of your hands as hooks. Make your back muscles do the work, pulling your elbows down and back as your torso ascends. Pause briefly at the top, squeezing your latissimus muscles. Then slowly lower back down to the start position.

▶ **CHECK IT!** Don't bounce or jerk. Keep your knees pointing toward the floor throughout the movement.

If you find chin-ups too difficult, or too easy, substitute this exercise with wide-grip pull-downs (chapter 10).

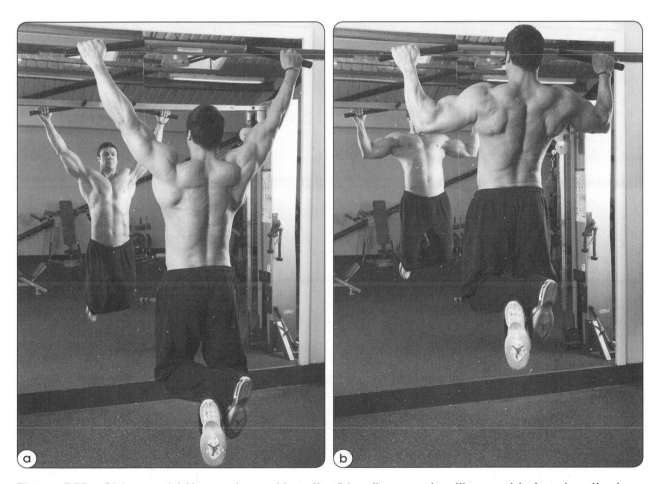

Figure 7.11 Chin-up: *(a)* Hang at arms' length; *(b)* pull upward until your chin touches the bar.

BACK

Barbell Row

Stand with feet about hip-width apart. Pick up a barbell with a shoulder-width grip. Tilt your upper body forward at the waist, making a 45-degree angle to the floor (figure 7.12*a*). Keep your lower back straight and head up. Begin the repetition by pulling the bar upward until it touches your upper abdomen (figure 7.12*b*). Pause briefly at the top, contracting your back muscles. Slowly return the weight to the straight-arm start position. This exercise can be performed with an overhand grip (palms turned down) or reverse underhand grip (palms turned up).

▶ **CHECK IT!**   Do not round your lower spine; avoid jerking up with your body.

Variations of the row exercise, such as seated rows (chapter 10) and dumbbell rows (chapter 14), are less strenuous on the lower back.

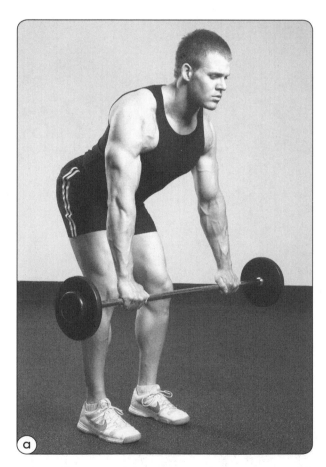 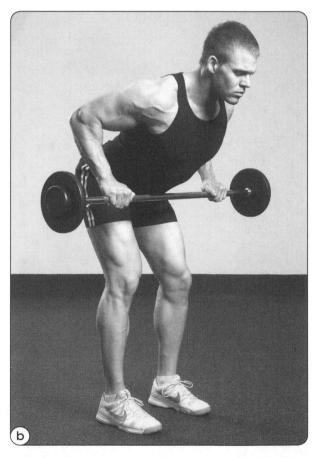

Figure 7.12   Barbell row: *(a)* Grip the barbell, torso angled to the floor; *(b)* lift the weight to your upper abdomen.

Barbell Curl

Stand upright holding a barbell at arms' length in front of you (figure 7.13a). Your hands should be shoulder-width apart in an underhand (palms up) grip. Curl the weight up by bending your arms at the elbows (figure 7.13b). Keep your elbows at your sides and your back straight. There should be little, if any, movement at the shoulder. Pause for one second at the top of the lift, keeping the bar at about chest level. Lower the bar slowly to the start position. Pause momentarily at the bottom of the lift, then repeat.

▶ **CHECK IT!** To reduce stress at the elbows, avoid excessively wide or narrow grips on the bar.

To keep tension on the biceps, stop a few degrees short of full elbow extension at the bottom, and don't let the bar rest on your upper thighs. There should be no backward or forward motion of your torso. You can also do this exercise on a biceps curl machine.

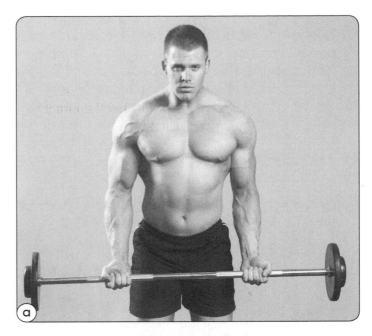

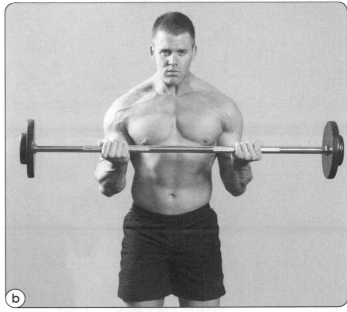

Figure 7.13 Barbell curl: (a) Stand holding the barbell; (b) curl the weight.

Incline Leg Raise

Adjust an abdominal bench to a 30-degree angle in relation to the floor. Lie supine with your head up. Hold the bench behind your head to stabilize your torso (figure 7.14a). From the start position, raise your legs at the hips. As you pull your thighs toward your chest, keep your knees slightly bent and your legs together. Tighten your lower abs as your hips bend. Stop before your thighs touch your chest, and hold the contracted position for one second (figure 7.14b). Then slowly lower your legs under control. Stop before your heels contact the bench (or the ground) to keep tension on the abdominal muscles. Hold in the bottom position momentarily, then repeat.

▶ **CHECK IT!** Position the bench at a steeper incline to increase the resistance.

You can also do leg raises while lying supine on a flat exercise bench. Variations of this exercise are described in chapters 10 and 14.

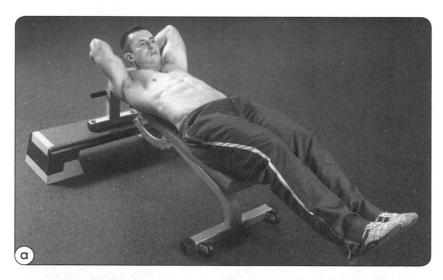

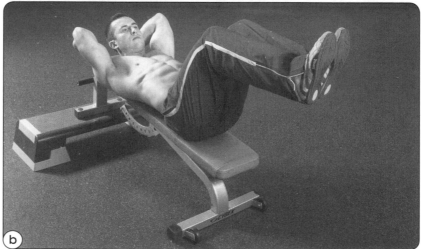

Figure 7.14 Incline leg raise: (a) Lie back on an incline bench; (b) lift legs toward chest.

Cutting Body Fat

In part III, you'll learn the best methods for cutting body fat. Building muscles is one thing; seeing them is another. Get the skinny on body fat in chapter 8, and learn the best weapons to torch your fat stores with extreme prejudice. That lean, mean, muscle machine will be yours, maybe sooner than you think. In chapter 9, you'll discover 12 simple steps toward gaining a lean advantage to optimize your body's fat-burning potential. The body fat blitz program in chapter 10 is tailored to melt away fat and get you that lean body look.

Lean Muscle Training

Building your muscles is one thing; being able to see them is another. What's the point in owning a set of strong, shapely muscles if you can't see them? It's like having a mint-condition vintage car that never leaves the garage. In the space between your skin and the underlying muscle lies a layer of fat. Fat owns that space; we rent it. Unless your body fat percentage is 10 percent or lower, that insulating layer of lard will obscure your hard-earned muscle mass.

The human body contains 20 to 30 billion fat cells. As well as providing a layer of insulation from the cold, body fat serves as an energy savings account; instead of money, the currency in this account is calories. The more calories you feed into the bank, the bigger the account gets.

Fat is a potent source of energy. Each gram of fat contains nine calories, compared with four calories per gram of protein or carbohydrate. So it's understandable that our bodies prefer to invest energy funds in a fat account. Fat storage is a survival mechanism; the swollen fat cells provide a savings account of calories to draw on during lean times. Fat cells are also resilient—they love to stick around and hate to get too small.

Not all fat is the same. A fat cell's precise qualities vary according to which fat deposit in the body it resides in. Fat from the belly, for instance, will lose and gain lipids more quickly than fat from the thighs and buttocks. When you're ridding your body of lard, the thighs and buttocks are the last areas that shed fat. In many people, these stubborn fat deposits won't disappear until body fat percentage slides below 6 percent.

So, how do you get rid of body fat and deflate that spare tire of blubber? You must stop feeding excess calories into the savings account. Stop making deposits, and start making withdrawals. When you withdraw calories from the savings account, the fat cells shrink in size, and their mass decreases.

In the fight against flab, the points on the scorecard are calories. Calories are the units of energy contained in food and are a measure of how much energy your body uses. When you consume more calories each day than you actually need, the excess is put into storage, and your body fat savings account grows. On the other hand, if you don't consume enough calories each day, the deficit is taken from savings—you burn body fat to provide the extra energy.

Each pound of body fat contains 3,500 calories. If your average daily calorie intake is 2,000 calories, you'd have to starve yourself for two days to lose that pound of fatty flesh. Even if you starved yourself for a week, theoretically omitting 2,000 calories per day, you'd lose only four pounds (1.8 kg) of body fat.

Starving out the army of fat cells is a tough battle to win. The good news is that we have a secret weapon—exercise. Exercise requires energy. To provide this energy, your body taps into its fat reserves. Exercise forces fat cells to give up their ammunition, their calorie stores. As the fat cells lose lipids, they shrink in size and decrease in volume.

Remember that losing fat depends on the balance between calories consumed and calories used. To shrink the fat cells, you either consume fewer calories, burn more calories, or both. As the fat melts away, your muscles come out to play, visible for all to see.

CALORIE-CRUNCHING TACTICS

The exercise of choice in the fight against fat is aerobic, or cardiorespiratory (cardio), exercise. The term *aerobic* indicates that the process requires oxygen. Aerobic exercise requires continuous movement with minimal resistance to stimulate the heart and lungs and expend calories—in other words, cardiorespiratory endurance exercise. Low-intensity, long-duration activities such as walking, jogging, and cycling are examples of cardiorespiratory exercise.

In building an effective aerobic program, you need to address several questions. How long should the activity last? How hard should you work? Which type of exercise is best? How many calories will you burn? How often should you perform the activity? When's the best time to do cardio? Let's discuss these questions in turn.

The duration of the exercise is important. To get an adequate training effect from aerobic activity, 20 to 30 minutes of continuous exercise is required. This is the minimum amount of time you should spend on cardio. If you want to maintain muscle size, don't exceed 60 minutes of cardio exercise. Longer periods of exercise are an endurance challenge, and your muscle framework will evolve into that of an endurance athlete. For fat burning, regular short bursts of cardio are superior to infrequent bouts of extended duration.

As a rule, the intensity of the cardio exercise (how hard you work) should be as high as you can make it. In other words, work as hard as you can for the 30-minute period. The harder you work, the more calories you burn. It's a mistake to assume that your half hour of cardio is a casual stroll. If you're not breathing heavy or breaking into a sweat, you're probably not working hard enough. You can tell the people who are exercising hard during cardio—they're not reading or talking!

If you have trouble judging your intensity level, here is a calculation that might help. Calculate your maximum heart rate by subtracting your age from 220. Multiply this figure by .7. This number is your target heart rate, which is 70 percent of the maximum heart rate for someone your age. For example, the target heart rate for a 30-year-old would be 133 (220 − 30 = 190; 190 × .7 = 133). This means that the target heart rate for a 30-year-old engaging in cardio activity is at least 130 beats per minute (70 percent of the estimated maximum heart rate of 190 beats per minute). Monitor your heart rate by feeling the pulse at your wrist and timing it over one minute using a watch. Eventually, you'll get to know how hard you should work to achieve your target heart rate without needing to constantly check

Heart Rate:
Can I measure my heart rate without a heart rate monitor?

Yes, timing your pulse using a wristwatch is a simple and reliable method. Here's how you do it. Locate the *radial* pulse at your wrist by turning your palm up and pressing lightly over the thumb side of your wrist with the index and middle fingers of the other hand. Count the number of beats over 15 seconds, then multiply this figure by 4 to calculate your pulse rate per minute. For example, if you count 30 beats of your pulse during 15 seconds, your heart rate is 120 beats per minute (30×4). I don't recommend monitoring the *carotid* pulse in your neck because it can restrict blood supply to your brain—not so good when you are exercising!

When it comes to choosing a cardio exercise, personal preference is the key factor. There are many different types to chose from. Outdoor activities include walking, jogging, and cycling. Indoor activities include riding a stationary bike, running on a treadmill, walking on a stair climber or elliptical trainer, or swimming in the pool. You're more likely to do the exercise effectively and regularly if you enjoy the activity. If you like variety, try different activities on different days of the week.

What determines how many calories you burn? The larger you are and the harder you work, the more calories you burn. Many factors play a part, such as your size, effort, muscles involved, fitness, amount of body fat, and movement efficiency as well as environmental conditions such as weather. With all these influences, accurately predicting how many calories you burn during your activities can be tough. However, you can make a useful approximation based on body weight. To help with your exercise program, look at the calorie-burning chart I've compiled for you (table 8.1).

Table 8.1 Calorie Burning Chart

Activity	Calories*
Jogging (6 mph; 10 km/h)	4.2
Jumping rope	3.8
Swimming	3.5
Cycling (10 mph; 16 km/h)	2.8
In-line skating	2.6
Walking (3 mph; 5 km/h)	2.4
Weight training	2.0

*Multiply this number by your body weight in pounds to calculate the calories burned per hour.

it. Many cardio machines have built-in heart rate monitors. You also can note the speed gauge. For example, 100 rpm on the stationary bike should put your heart rate in the target range. The worst-case scenario is that you become so obsessed with checking your pulse that you're not paying enough attention to the exercise.

Using a calorie burning chart is easy (table 8.1). Let's say you weigh 200 pounds (91 kg). The approximate number of calories burned during one hour of weight training would be 200 × 2.0, or 400 calories. The calories burned during a 30-minute weight-training session would be 200. For comparison, 30 minutes of walking would burn 240 calories, cycling would burn 280 calories, and jogging would burn 420 calories.

In general, *standing* weight-bearing exercises are more demanding than *seated* non-weight-bearing activities. For example, jogging burns nearly twice as many calories per minute as does cycling. The calorie expenditure using most cardio *machines* is similar. When you compare the upright versus recumbent bike, there is not a great deal of difference. Functionally, sitting upright is a more effective cycling posture, whereas the recumbent position can stress your lower back and restrict your breathing capacity. My recommendation is to go with personal preference—if you enjoy the exercise, you're more likely to do it.

Remember that these calculations are only estimates, but it's always true that the harder you work, the more calories you burn. An intense half hour of weights in which you lift as much weight as possible with minimum rest between sets will burn more than the estimated value. The key to burning more calories during a weight-training session is reducing the rest interval between sets and exercises. If you'd prefer to make a quicker calculation of the number of calories burned, use these estimates for one minute of exercise:

Running: 12 calories per minute

Cycling: 8 calories per minute

Walking: 6 calories per minute

Weight training: 6 calories per minute

Remember that this minute-by-minute estimation does not take into account your body weight. In fact, for every pound (.5 kg) of lean muscle you pack onto your frame, you'll burn an additional 30 calories per day at rest.

Aerobic exercise should be done two or three days per week, preferably on the days you don't train with weights. Cardio and weight training serve different purposes. With weight training, you're aiming to grow muscle size and strength. During cardio, you're trying to expend calories to burn fat. When you combine cardio and weight training in the same workout, you'll still burn fat, but muscle growth might suffer. Personally, I like to alternate between a weight-training

Rowing: What is your opinion on the rowing machine?

Exercise selection usually comes down to personal preference or fitness goals. Rowing is a demanding whole-body exercise that ranks highly in terms of effort and calorie expenditure. But it is especially hard on the back, arms, and legs. If you lift a lot of weights, selecting the rowing machine for cardio might be counterproductive and lead to overtraining your back and arms. Bodybuilders typically use cardio exercises that burn body fat without losing muscle mass. When you exercise on a stationary bike, treadmill, or elliptical trainer, the muscles of your upper body get some respite.

workout one day and a cardio session the next. If you prefer to combine the two types of exercise during one workout, do the weights session before the cardio.

The fat-burning effect of cardio is greatest if you perform the exercise first thing in the morning on an empty stomach. Since you have fasted for eight hours overnight, your body's supply of glucose energy is low. As a result, you're more likely to tap into fat reserves for energy. Whatever time of day you perform cardio, you can still achieve a similar effect by not eating for at least two hours before exercise. Furthermore, your body continues to burn stored energy even after you stop exercising. To maximize this effect, wait an hour after cardio before eating. Remember that the goal of low-intensity, calorie-crunching cardio is to lose body fat, not to generate an anabolic effect.

When it comes to choosing your own personal exercise prescription, be guided by your individual body type and goals. If you are an ectomorph, your primary goal is to gain muscle mass. Your particular focus lies with weight training rather than cardio, and you should select the mass generator program discussed in chapter 7. On the other hand, an endomorph needs to focus on fat loss. For this purpose, you'll need to include some calorie-crunching cardio; you should select the body fat blitz program covered in chapter 10.

HIGH-SPEED CARDIO

If you fancy a change from the standard low-intensity cardio session on the exercise bike, treadmill, or elliptical trainer, why not try interval sprint training? Recent research has shown that high-intensity interval training (HIIT) consisting of short, lung-searing bouts of cardio is more effective than longer, steady-pace efforts on most cardio machines in the gym. Science suggests that HIIT is a more efficient way to burn fat while preserving muscle mass. What's more, HIIT also increases resting metabolism over the subsequent 24 hours. The only downside of HIIT is that it is best performed outdoors and therefore falls into the weather-permitting category of cardio. Unless, of course, you enjoy the prospect of a Rocky Balboa session of cardio stomping through the snow! Two sample interval sprint training routines are shown in table 8.2. These routines are not for the faint of heart. Before each workout, take 5 to 10 minutes to warm up. Make sure you stretch appropriately to ensure your leg muscles' range of motion is sufficient for sprinting. And remember that the best location for sprint training is an actual running track.

Table 8.2 High-Intensity Interval Training Cardio Routines

10-second sprint training	Sprint-to-stride training
10 sec sprint + 1 min jog Repeat for a total of 20 min.	30 sec sprint-to-stride + 1 min walk Repeat 3 times. Cool down with a 2 min walk. Repeat cycle 3 times. Total time = 25 min
This is a continuous-motion interval. Do not stop between sprints. Ease into the 1 min jogs, then ramp back up into the sprints.	With the sprint-to-stride workout, maintain your pace for as long as possible, then as you fatigue, slow down to a walking pace.

SIX-PACK SECRETS

During my decade as a fitness magazine columnist, the question I was most frequently asked was, "How do I get a six-pack?" Everybody wants a set of defined abdominal muscles. The trouble is that the misconceptions surrounding how to attain a tight midsection leave many people struggling to find methods that work. You see, you can perform as many sit-ups as you like or work on crunches until you're blue in the face, but until you ditch that spare tire around your waist, you'll never see a chiseled set of abs, period. If you want abs that look as if they were etched out of stone, you have to carve off the fat that covers them.

There is no simple "ab-solution," and there isn't a magic pill, but I do have a six-pack prescription for phenomenal abdominals. The process consists of several simple steps that, when combined, work like magic.

1. **Do your cardio.** Perform 30 minutes of cardio at least three times a week. During each session, you'll burn around 200 calories. What's more, if you do your cardio first thing in the morning on an empty stomach, you'll burn up to three times more fat. Because you haven't eaten all night, your sugar levels are low, which makes early morning the optimal time for fat loss. When you perform cardio in this state, your fat stores are used as fuel.

2. **Eat six small meals a day.** If you eat smaller meals, your stomach can reduce in size, and you'll feel satisfied with less food. This helps prevent that bloated belly look. Consuming smaller meals every three hours provides a constant supply of energy and prevents hunger pangs.

3. **Reduce your calorie intake.** If you burn more calories each day than you consume, you'll lose body fat. The best way to reduce calorie intake is to cut down your consumption of dietary fat. Each gram of fat contains nine calories, which is double the amount contained in either a gram of protein or carbohydrate. Be sure to stick with low-fat or nonfat food products.

4. **Increase your protein intake.** Protein is less likely to cause body fat deposits than either carbohydrate or fat. The larger the protein component of your diet, the more effective your powers of fat burning. Consume 1 gram of protein per pound of body weight daily to feed your muscles and keep your metabolism elevated.

5. **Cut back on carbohydrate.** Dietary carbohydrate is essential for energy, but eating more carbohydrate than you need will feed your body fat. When your carbohydrate stores are filled, excess sugar is converted to fat. If you restrict your carbohydrate intake, your body is forced to burn fat stores for energy. To achieve this effect, carbohydrate should account for less than 50 percent of your total calorie intake each day. When choosing carbohydrate, pick foods with a low glycemic index, such as the complex carbohydrates in brown (whole-grain) rice, potatoes, and pasta. Keep your consumption of high-glycemic simple sugar, such as bananas, fruit juice, white bread, and white rice, to a minimum.

6. **Drink water, not soda.** For health reasons, it's important to keep your body well hydrated. But if you satisfy your thirst with soda, milk, fruit juice, or alcohol, you're consuming extra calories. It's easy to forget that an 8-ounce (240 ml) beverage can contain 100 to 200 calories. If you want to keep the fat off, water is the way to go. Consume at least one gallon (nearly 4 L) of water per day.

7. **Work your abdominals.** Everybody has abdominal muscles. The problem is that they hide under a layer of body fat. Targeting your waist with specific abdominal exercises is important if you want a six-pack. Still, as I've mentioned, it doesn't matter how many exercises you do if your abdominals are covered in fat because no one is going to see them. In fact, your body fat percentage must be below 10 percent before you'll witness any visible benefit from abdominal exercises. But even if you can't see the individual muscles, a toned and tight abdomen prevents your belly from protruding. Choose a series of exercises that work all areas of the abdomen. Sit-ups or crunches target the upper abdominals, leg raises work the lower abdominals, and a twisting exercise tones the obliques. Perform three sets of each exercise two or three times each week.

8. **The more lean muscle you have, the more calories you'll burn on a daily basis.** For every pound of lean muscle you add, you'll burn an extra 30 calories per day at rest. As you know, more calories burned equals more fat lost.

9. **Try a fat burner.** Weight-loss supplements containing active ingredients such as caffeine, Garcinia cambogia, green tea, or hoodia can assist in promoting fat loss. These agents are thought to suppress appetite and elevate your body's metabolic rate so you burn more calories. Make sure you read the product label carefully, and if you have any medical conditions, check with your doctor before using fat-loss supplements. For more information on fat burners, see chapter 13.

10. **Be dedicated.** You won't get a six-pack overnight. If you follow all the steps, you can lose a pound or two of body fat each week, and within a month you'll witness progress. There's no substitute for dedication and discipline. Be patient, stick with the plan, and soon you'll have your very own six-pack.

The most important exercise to develop a slim waist is cardio, but what you eat is equally important. If you have another look at the 10 steps, you'll see that 5 of them involve changes to your diet. So, in addition to burning calories, you must address calorie consumption. Chapter 2 teaches you all the essential nutrition knowledge. In chapter 9, we'll discuss additional skills for gaining a lean advantage.

Gaining a Lean Advantage

Your body is a biological environment. When that environment is anabolic, your body tends to gain weight. Conversely, when that environment is catabolic, your body tends to lose weight. The problem with being too catabolic is that you lose muscle mass as well as body fat. So if you want to shed body fat but maintain muscle, you need to tease your body's environment in the right direction by gaining a lean advantage. You can turn up the heat in your fat-burning furnace with the following 12 steps:

1. Count on the three Cs.
2. Keep on moving.
3. Use the fat-burning window.
4. Maintain hormone balance.
5. Use supplements to help shed fat.
6. Try speed workouts.
7. Watch your waistline.
8. Sleep more for less fat.
9. Think before you drink.
10. Choose the right diet.
11. Forget spot reducing.
12. Suit your body type.

In this chapter, we look at each of these steps in more detail and incorporate them into a strategic fat-shedding program.

COUNT ON THE THREE CS

The keys to fat loss are the three Cs: calories, carbohydrate, and cardio. We have already discussed the importance of the calorie count and nutrient profile in your diet (chapter 2) and established the calorie-crunching powers of exercise (chapter 8). To lose body fat, you must be in a *negative* caloric balance by burning more calories than you consume. To achieve this, you either increase your calorie expenditure with exercise, or you decrease your calorie intake with diet—or you combine both tactics. Being in a negative caloric balance forces your body to burn fat stores to generate extra energy.

When planning your diet, the first thing to do is estimate your maintenance daily calorie requirement (body weight in pounds × 10, or your body weight in kilograms × 22) then subtract 10 percent from this amount to figure out your daily calorie intake for fat-burning purposes. This calculation deprives your body of 10 percent fewer calories than it would need to maintain energy production during the day. To match this energy deficit, your body generates the extra calories by burning body fat. In addition to calculating the calorie count, you need to decide which nutrients those calories will come from. To encourage fat loss, I recommend that you reduce the ratio of carbohydrate in your diet. The nutrient proportion should be high protein (50 percent), moderate carbohydrate (40 percent), and low fat (10 percent). You'll find specific calculations together with sample meal plans for fat loss in chapter 10.

It's important to monitor your progress using a weighing scale. If your weight is not decreasing as the weeks go by, then clearly you are not in a negative caloric balance, and you must be consuming a surplus of calories. Decrease your calorie intake by another 5 percent each week until your weight starts moving in the right direction. This *gradual* decrease in calories avoids a drastic drop that could lead to losing muscle as well as fat.

If you reach a plateau, or sticking point, in your body weight or body fat percentage, you have three possible solutions using the rule of the three Cs:

1. **Cardio:** Increase the amount of cardio by extending the duration of aerobic exercise or adding extra sessions to your weekly schedule. You could also try high-speed cardio using interval sprint training (see chapter 8), which affords a more effective fat burn compared with most cardio machines.

2. **Calories:** Reduce your calorie intake by omitting your cheat day, reducing the number of meals you eat, or subtracting 5 to 10 percent increments from your daily total calorie intake.

3. **Carbohydrate:** Cut back on carbohydrate by eliminating carbohydrate foods from your last meal of the day or gradually reducing carbohydrate portions so that the nutrient ratio of your diet moves toward 60 percent protein, 30 percent carbohydrate, and 10 percent fat.

KEEP ON MOVING

Humans are creatures of habit. Given the choice, we stick with the same routine day in, day out. If you have a sedentary job, you probably expend only the minimum amount of calories per day when you're not working out. On any given day, you leave home, slump in the car, and drive to work. Then you take the elevator up to your office, sit at your desk all day, and then drive back home. The bottom line is that your metabolic rate rarely fluctuates above baseline. If you want to lose weight, you've got to *move* more—simple. Your options include walking, stair climbing, cycling, and jogging. Walking for 30 minutes burns roughly 200 calories, depending on speed, body weight, etc. Take a moment and think how you can modify your daily routine to incorporate some incidental cardio. Distance permitting, you could walk or cycle to work. Do a little exercise during your break. Climb the stairs in your office building instead of taking the elevator. Strategically including a little incidental exercise here and there can make a big difference in your daily calorie expenditure. And burning an extra few hundred calories a day elevates your basal metabolic rate and makes a substantial contribution to fat loss.

USE THE FAT-BURNING WINDOW

Probably the best time of day to burn fat is first thing in the morning. After an overnight sleep, your body is starved of nutrients because you haven't eaten anything for about eight hours. Your body's supply of ready energy is low, so you are more likely to tap into your fat reserves. In fact, you could burn up to three times more fat when you train before breakfast. It's also worth remembering that your body continues to burn fat stores after you stop exercising. So to maximize this delayed fat-burning effect, wait an hour after working out before you eat. If you combine your weights and cardio sessions in one workout, lift weights before you perform cardio.

MAINTAIN HORMONE BALANCE

Testosterone and growth hormone have powerful anabolic actions that build muscle *and* reduce body fat. It follows then that if both these hormones are abundant in your body, you will create an environment that promotes lean muscle mass, fat burning, and fat loss. Now, exercise is a paradox of sorts. Short, intense bouts of exercise boost anabolic hormone levels, whereas too much exercise makes the body antianabolic, or catabolic. Excessive amounts of cardio can actually reduce your levels of testosterone and growth hormone, adversely affecting your fat-burning capability. As such, a decline in anabolic hormones contributes to fat accumulation and diminished energy, strength, and muscle mass. So the trick is to perform enough exercise to promote fat loss but not to overdo it. It's better to do 30 minutes of cardio regularly rather than an hour or more of cardio sporadically. You want to stimulate, not annihilate, your body's fat-burning capability. Enhance your body's natural production of anabolic hormones with regular short bouts of intense exercise, a high-protein diet, and adequate sleep. As your body fat drops, your levels of anabolic hormones will increase, and vice versa.

USE SUPPLEMENTS TO HELP SHED FAT

Nutritional supplements can assist in your quest to lose body fat. Obviously, there are the fat burners. But other supplements can be useful in helping you control your calorie intake. If you work and are away from home for eight hours a day, it is difficult to feed your body with a regular dose of quality nutrients in the right amounts. And it's not easy to prepare several calorie-controlled meals each day. Even so, if you want to shed fat with all your hard work in the gym, you must fuel your body appropriately. And this is where quality nutritional supplements are useful.

Meal-replacement formulas are a convenient substitute for meals of solid food. A high-protein and low-fat meal-replacement drink is a healthier and often cheaper alternative to a fat-loaded meal of fast food. A quality meal-replacement product should provide a detailed list of the nutrients, making it easy to accurately control your calorie intake. Let's say the whole sachet contains 300 calories, but you want just 150 calories. All you need to do is mix *half* the sachet with water in a blender.

When dieting, you might find that meal-replacement supplements contain more carbohydrate than your diet allows. When partitioning nutrients in a high-protein, low-carbohydrate ratio, protein-only supplements are particularly useful. Whether it's a powdered protein preparation or a ready-to-drink protein formula, a 30-gram drink is likely to contain less than 200 calories. If you want to add a measured amount of carbohydrate to the protein drink, you can add some fruit. Low-carbohydrate protein bars are also a useful addition to your lunch box.

Multivitamin and mineral supplements are an excellent addition to any nutrition plan to prevent dietary deficiencies. If you are restricting your intake with a reduced-calorie diet, it may be difficult to ensure that you are meeting your required daily intake of essential vitamins and minerals.

That brings us to the subject of weight-loss supplements and fat burners. These products can increase the body's natural fat-burning potential. They work via a process called thermogenesis, causing a natural elevation in your metabolic rate, allowing you to theoretically burn more calories while at rest and during exercise. The more calories burned, the greater the weight loss. The active ingredients in fat-loss supplements are typically natural extracts thought to support thermogenesis, enhance fat oxidation, suppress appetite, and increase calorie expenditure. Currently, such ingredients include caffeine, Garcinia cambogia (hydroxycitric acid), green tea, and hoodia. Fat-loss agents work best when combined with a low-calorie, low-fat diet and regular aerobic exercise. These products are discussed in more detail in chapter 13.

TRY SPEED WORKOUTS

One of my secrets for shredding up lies in the *speed* of my weights workout. I'm not talking about rep speed but the speed with which I proceed between sets and exercises with minimum downtime. From the moment I step foot in the gym, I'm pretty much exercising nonstop for 30 to 40 minutes. During speed workouts, I train alone, have my personal stereo on, and am completely focused—no talking, no reading, and no making notes in a workout journal. As usual, I perform each rep of every exercise in a slow, controlled, precise manner, with as much weight as I can safely handle for 8 to 12 reps. But I go from set to set and move from exercise to exercise with virtually no rest at all. I utilize a lot of machines so that I do not waste time changing weights or loading bars. If I do rest, it's no longer than 15 to 30 seconds. This type of calorie-crunching speed workout is intense. Basically, you'll get a 40-minute workout completed in less than 30 minutes. It's a major calorie burn, but you'll be stimulating muscle growth at the same time. And remember, working the bigger muscles (legs, chest, back) burns more calories than working the smaller muscle groups (biceps, triceps, calves).

Supersets: What's the theory behind supersets, and are they effective?

A *superset* involves performing two different exercises back to back without a rest interval. When you combine more than two exercises in this way, then the sequence becomes a *giant* set. The theory is that the muscle fibers exhausted by the first set do not have time to recover, so during the subsequent set(s) the muscle must recruit even more fibers to lift the weight. Shortening the rest interval between sets affords three main benefits: It (1) stimulates more muscle fibers, (2) raises the intensity, and (3) burns more calories. Hence, supersets are an effective way to build muscle and burn fat at the same time. What's more, because you are performing more work in less time, the duration of your workout session will be shorter.

WATCH YOUR WAISTLINE

Reducing your waistline is one thing, and building your abdominal and oblique muscles is another. They are opposing objectives. The size of your waist is determined by three anatomical factors, namely hip bones, body fat, and abdominal muscles. You cannot change the width of your hip bones since that is determined by genetics. What you do have control over is the amount of body fat on your belly and the condition of your abdominal muscles. However, if you *build* the muscular wall of your abdomen, then your waist will become *thicker* not thinner. Just like any muscle group, the abdominals and obliques will grow in size when exercised with weights. And bigger obliques offset the chest-to-waist size differential, giving the appearance of a blocky waist. So, if your primary goal is to reduce your waistline, you should focus on burning body fat, not building big obliques. A smaller waist means eating less and exercising more. In other words, your main strategy should involve diet and cardio. Now, if you wish to tone your oblique muscles, there are several exercises to choose from including twisting sit-ups, oblique crunches, and side bends. But in order to avoid increasing your waist size, I'd recommend performing high reps using body weight or minimal added resistance.

SLEEP MORE FOR LESS FAT

Stay up late and crawl out of bed too early, and you'll get what's coming to you: baggy eyes, low energy, a foul mood, and maybe some extra body fat. Chronic lack of sleep may be one reason many people are getting broad in the belly. Sleep deprivation increases cortisol levels, resulting in water retention, and recent research has also discovered that going without sleep elevates blood levels of an appetite-stimulating hormone, called *ghrelin*, and decreases levels of an appetite-suppressing hormone, known as *leptin*. The likely net effect is an increase in appetite. During the study, volunteer subjects who slept the least had the most ghrelin and the least leptin. For those who slept the longest, the results were reversed. Scientists also found that the subjects with the least sleep had a higher body mass index (BMI), a measure of being overweight. What's more, the volunteers rated themselves as significantly more hungry, especially for high-calorie food, when they had been deprived of sleep. So it seems that lack of sleep induces hunger.

No doubt, a good night's sleep makes good sense. However, sleep is not necessarily the only answer. If you are unable to get sufficient sleep, at least six hours, you've got to watch what you're eating during those extra hours when you are up and about. If you're tired, it's very tempting to raid the refrigerator for easy-to-eat junk. Late at night, you'd best stay away from high-carbohydrate, fatty foods that tend to bloat your waistline.

THINK BEFORE YOU DRINK

Just like the chorus of a catchy pop song, the phrase *think before you drink* is a repetitive hook throughout this book. The reason: People tend to turn a blind eye to the concept of *liquid* calories. If a liquid has color, flavor, or bubbles, chances are it contains calories. The only liquid that *definitely* has zero calories is unadulterated still water. So, let's take this opportunity to discuss two popular calorific drinks, namely alcohol and flavored coffees.

Now, I'm sure most adults can testify to the unpleasant aftereffects of too much alcohol. But in addition to the postbinge hangover, there's something else that fitness folk should be concerned about—consuming a calorie-loaded cocktail that kills your conditioning. Newsflash: Alcohol can be a big problem for fat-conscious bodybuilders. Why? There are several reasons. Alcohol adversely affects exercise performance and recovery. It can cause dehydration and nutrition deficiencies. Alcohol is also a source of unnecessary calories. It doesn't matter how meticulous you are with your diet, if you're drinking alcohol every day, you won't get ultra-lean. What's more, alcohol interferes with the body's ability to burn fat. Your body uses alcohol as an energy source rather than deriving it from stored fat, so your body holds on to fat, contributing to that beer belly. Think before you drink, and check out these facts:

1. A regular beer has about 150 calories.
2. A six-ounce (180 ml) glass of red wine has 120 calories.
3. A margarita can contain 450 calories.
4. Partygoers who drink a Red Bull with vodka slurp down 250 calories.
5. Many cocktails contain more calories than a double cheeseburger.
6. Drinking a glass of wine every day adds up to an extra 40,000 calories per year.

You may also be tempted by the lure of a refreshing jolt of iced java. The trendy java huts have been busy creating new chilled recipes to tempt our taste buds during the hot summer months. But for the consumer, there's a hefty price to pay. These cold, flavored coffee drinks not only cost an arm and a leg but also pack a hefty caloric punch. How many calories? Well, make sure you are sitting down, because you're in for quite a shock. Check these data out. First up, let's evaluate a medium-size 16-ounce (480 ml) cup of black coffee. As you might expect, this standard favorite contains only 10 calories from a couple of grams of carbohydrate. Next, a 16-ounce cup of cappuccino bumps the calorie count up to around 150 calories on account of the steamed milk. Now here's the shocker, a 16-ounce serving of one of those new blended iced coffee drinks contains nearly

300 calories. And when you add whipped cream to that drink, it delivers a whopping 430 calories with a massive 16 grams of fat. Yep, you read that right. Quench your thirst with this baby, and you'll gulp down almost 500 calories. If you're looking for a fast-acting weight-gain supplement, this is it, my friend. Sadly, you probably won't find these nutrition facts on display in the coffee shops—and that ought to be a red flag for any calorie-conscious bodybuilder. Personally, I think that any 500-calorie drink should come with a health warning on the cup! If you want anything that resembles an abdominal six-pack, you'd best stay clear of the java with a hidden jolt of calories. You could request that your drink be made less calorific by using nonfat milk, but even then you'll still get a drink that tops out at around 200 calories. If you are serious about losing fat, choose a chilled ready-to-drink can of protein.

CHOOSE THE RIGHT DIET

No doubt, there are many paths up the same mountain. Everyone, it seems, is jumping on the fat-loss wagon these days, inventing a diet, writing a book, and selling a supplement. You've got the Hollywood diet, the South Beach diet, the Atkins diet, and so on, and just about every possible idea is being recommended: high fat, low carbohydrate, this, that, and the other. You've got to realize that most mainstream diets are aimed at the general public, those legions of overweight people who overeat and don't exercise. The average Joe is not going to sign up for a diet that is too strict or requires some serious dietary discipline. The diet for a bodybuilder who wishes to get lean is very different from all those other diet plans. You're looking at a diet designed to drop your body fat into single digits while maintaining a significant amount of muscle mass. You're also talking about a diet that aims to achieve these goals as quickly as possible.

A bodybuilder's diet is also different from an athlete's diet, where the primary goal is to provide energy to perform without losing fat. The key is to choose the diet that's right for you. If you simply want to lose that tubby tire of lard around your waist and be able to wear your old pants again, then any diet book may help. If you're looking to boost athletic performance, then research sport-specific dieting. But if you want to be lean and muscular, you should follow a bodybuilding-type diet plan.

FORGET SPOT REDUCING

Almost everybody experiences problems with stubborn areas of fat. Why? Because not all body fat is the same. A fat cell's precise qualities vary according to which part of the body it resides in. There are also genetic differences in your body's preferred locations for fat storage. For instance, fat from the belly tends to lose and gain lipids more quickly than fat from the thighs and buttocks, where fat cells are resilient and like to stick around. So, when you're ridding your body of lard, these stubborn spots are the last areas that shed fat. The only way to spot reduce specific fat zones is to undergo liposuction surgery. If you want to zap those hard-to-slim-down spots naturally, you've got to reduce your body fat percentage to 10 percent or less! Remember, losing fat depends on the balance between calories consumed and calories used. To shed stubborn fat, you must *maintain* a negative calorie balance—until you get the job done.

SUIT YOUR BODY TYPE

As discussed in chapter 4, the three basic body types are ectomorph, mesomorph, and endomorph. Each body type requires a different bodybuilding prescription. The endomorph body type tends to have a slow metabolism that stores unwanted extra calories, so an endomorph easily gains weight but struggles to lose body fat. The main goal for an endomorph is to burn off excess body fat, so his body-sculpting program must be prescribed with this in mind. The exercise program for an endomorph should include several cardio sessions per week. Weight training should be performed at a fast pace utilizing higher repetitions. When it comes to nutrition, a low-calorie diet is essential for an endomorph. To promote fat loss, daily calorie intake must be less than the daily calorie expenditure. And the nutrient ratio should be high in protein and low in fat, with a moderate amount of complex carbohydrate. Snacking and cheat days are best avoided if you are looking to get lean.

Once your body has shed its excess body fat, you can switch from a fat-loss program to a muscle-building regimen. However, if the endomorph shape is your default body type, you may have to incorporate a couple of cardio sessions in your workout plan to keep the fat from creeping back (see chapter 14).

Now that you know how to heat up your fat-burning furnace, you're ready to shed some serious body fat. In the next chapter we unveil your personal prescription for losing pounds of unwanted fat. Read on to discover the ultimate body fat blitz workout and a scientific diet that burns body fat with extreme prejudice.

Body Fat Blitz Program

In the last two chapters we focus on fat loss. We look at the calorie-crunching powers of exercise and establish the importance of the calorie count and nutrient profile in your diet. Now it's time to put these fat-burning theories into practice.

If you're looking to lose unwanted body fat quickly, this is the plan for you. I have combined a selection of resistance and aerobic exercises into a four-day workout routine that increases your metabolic rate and melts away your fat stores. To maximize calorie use, you'll perform between 10 and 15 repetitions of each weight-training exercise, keeping the rest interval between sets under 60 seconds. The fat-loss diet aims to create a daily calorie deficit so that the negative caloric balance forces your body to burn fat stores to provide energy.

PROGRAM OVERVIEW

The body fat blitz program is designed to burn body fat. To promote calorie burning, the weights program emphasizes higher reps with lower resistance. Perform three sets of each exercise, using weights equal to 60 to 70 percent of your one-rep maximum. After an initial warm-up set of 15 reps, increase the weight on your second set so that your muscles fatigue with 12 reps. Then, on the final set, add more weight, and squeeze out 10 reps to failure. To keep your heart rate elevated—and to burn more calories—keep your rest intervals short. Move through the workouts at a fast pace, taking only 30 to 60 seconds of rest between sets and exercises. Aim to complete each workout in 30 to 40 minutes.

Even though you're lifting lighter weights (60 to 70 percent of your one-rep max) with a higher repetition range, training to failure on the last set of 10 reps *will* stimulate muscle hypertrophy. And remember that for every pound of lean muscle you add to your body, you'll burn an extra 30 calories per day at rest. So training to failure, especially on the final work set, is your goal for each exercise. The more muscle you possess, the more calories you burn during a workout.

Workout Plan

The body fat blitz routine uses an upper body–lower body two-way split-training system combined with two cardio workouts. I'll explain how the schedule works. Session 1 works the entire upper body (chest, shoulders, back, arms). Session 2 consists of aerobic exercise and an abdominal workout. Session 3 works the lower body (quads, hamstrings, calves). Session 4 is another combined aerobic and abdominal workout.

The prime objective of this program is *lean* muscle mass. You're striving to burn calories and shed unwanted body fat. The two sessions per week of weight training will also build muscle. And by increasing your fat-free mass (muscle), you become more efficient at burning calories. Whether you burn 300 calories by lifting weights or cycling on a stationary bike, 300 calories is 300 calories. Although aerobic exercise doesn't increase muscle mass, your body recovers quickly after cardio, so you can use this form of calorie-burning exercise (every day if necessary) without worrying about overtraining.

During the weight-training sessions, you'll burn more calories by using unilateral (single-limb) training on selected exercises. By training one side at a time, you can rest one limb while the other works, so you won't need as much rest between sets. Each limb gets adequate rest, but your cardiorespiratory system gets less rest. Because you're training one side at a time, your workouts will take a little longer, but you'll be doing more work with less total rest and thus burning more

Unilateral Training

Working one side of your body at a time is known as single-limb, or unilateral training. Bodybuilders frequently turn upper body movements into one-arm exercises using dumbbells, cables, or machines. Training one side at a time works for nearly all muscle groups of the upper body, including biceps, triceps, deltoids, chest, lats, and forearms. Single-leg training is a little more difficult, but it will work for several exercises such as leg extensions, leg curls, leg presses, lunges, and calf raises. Unilateral training offers several benefits:

1. **Allows better contraction:** Working one limb allows you to focus entirely on one muscle, without distraction from the other limb. If all your effort is channeled into one muscle, you can make it work harder and achieve a better contraction. And during certain exercises, such as the one-arm biceps curl, the other (free) hand can assist with some forced reps.

2. **Improves symmetry:** Unilateral training is perfect for eliminating side-to-side muscle imbalances, promoting symmetry, and minimizing the size differences between your dominant and nondominant sides.

3. **Burns more calories:** Although your workouts may take a little longer, training one side at a time burns more calories. You can rest one limb while the other works, so you won't need as much rest between sets. You'll do more work with less total rest and therefore burn more calories.

4. **Useful during injury:** Unilateral training is useful when one limb is injured, allowing continued training of the noninjured limb. So, even though you're resting the injury, you can still get a workout. Furthermore, many of the strength gains and neural benefits of the exercising muscle are transferred to the nonexercising muscle of the opposite limb, which can speed recovery from injury.

calories. Examples of unilateral exercises included in this program are dumbbell curls, leg extensions, and leg curls.

Calorie-burning cardiorespiratory exercise is a key part of any fat-loss program. This continuous low-resistance exercise must be performed for at least 20 minutes to achieve an adequate training effect. Work hard enough to maintain your heart rate in the target zone—70 percent of your maximum heart rate. (Calculate your target heart rate by subtracting your age from 220 and then multiplying this figure by .7.)

The type of aerobic exercise you do is up to you. There are many indoor and outdoor activities to choose from, including walking, jogging, cycling, stair climbing, jumping rope, and swimming. It's more challenging if you vary the aerobic exercise, selecting a different activity for each cardio session. For example, cycle on a stationary bike during session 2, then walk or jog on the treadmill during session 4. Once you have completed 30 minutes of cardio, you'll do 10 minutes of abdominal exercises to round off the session. The exercises included in this program target all areas of your midsection—the upper and lower portions of your abs, the obliques, and the serratus muscles. Remember that any abdominal work will be *visibly* evident only if your body fat percentage is 10 percent or less.

Nutrition Plan

To lose body fat, burn more calories than you consume. Being in a negative caloric balance forces the body to burn fat stores to generate extra energy. Just how many calories should you consume each day during your fat-loss program? First, calculate your maintenance daily calorie requirement (body weight in pounds × 10, or body weight in kilograms × 22). Then subtract 10 percent from this amount to get your daily calorie intake for fat-burning purposes. In other words, you are depriving your body of 10 percent fewer calories than it needs for energy production on a daily basis. To meet this energy deficit, your body gets the extra calories by burning body fat.

The 1,600-calorie sample meal plan in table 10.1 is a rough guide for someone who weighs 180 pounds (82 kg). The daily calorie intake is equivalent to an 1,800-calorie maintenance value (180 pounds × 10) minus 10 percent, which brings the calorie total to 1,620 calories.

Next, decide which food sources your calories will come from. To promote fat loss, you'll need to cut back on the ratio of carbohydrate in your diet. Divide the nutrients as follows: 50 percent protein, 40 percent carbohydrate, and 10 percent fat.

Adjusting the sample meal plan to your weight is easy. As you might recall from chapter 2, 1 gram of protein is 4 calories, 1 gram of carbohydrate is 4 calories, and 1 gram of fat is 9 calories. Keeping the nutrient ratio at 50 percent protein and 40 percent carbohydrate, 100 calories equals 15 grams of protein (60 calories) plus 10 grams of carbohydrate (40 calories). To increase or decrease the calorie content to match your body weight, add or subtract these amounts from the sample meal plan.

Progression is essential if you want ongoing fat loss. Remember, as your body weight decreases, so will your estimated daily calorie intake by a factor of 10—10 calories per pound of body weight. For instance, when your body weight drops by five pounds (2.3 kg), you should decrease your daily calorie intake by 50 calories. Check your weight each week, and make the appropriate adjustment using table 10.2. This *gradual* decrease in calories avoids a drastic drop that could lead to losing muscle as well as fat.

Table 10.1   Body Fat Blitz Sample Meal Plan

Breakfast	Egg-white scramble: Mix five egg whites with 1 tbsp of nonfat milk. Cook in a nonstick pan coated with nonfat cooking spray. Serve on one piece of whole-wheat toast. Drink one cup of black coffee or water. Calories: 230 (see discussion in 14.1)
Midmorning snack	Meal-replacement drink: Mix one sachet of a meal-replacement powder with 12 oz (360 ml) cold water in a blender. Calories: 340
Lunch	Tuna meal: Drain one 6-oz (175 g) can of water-packed tuna and squeeze some lemon juice over it. Serve with a portion of steamed brown rice. Drink a glass of ice water. Calories: 300
Midafternoon snack	Protein drink: Mix one serving of protein powder with 4 oz (120 ml) water and 4 oz nonfat milk. Add one whole banana. Blend at high speed for 30 seconds. Calories: 240
Dinner	Chicken meal: Prepare a skinless chicken breast by squeezing lemon juice over it. Grill until cooked. Serve with a portion of steamed brown rice and spinach or broccoli. A tbsp of tomato ketchup is optional. Calories: 380
Late-evening snack	Eat half a low-carbohydrate protein bar. Calories: 150
Daily values (approximate)	Protein: 200 g (800 cal), 50% Carbohydrate: 160 g (640 cal), 40% Fat: 17 g (160 cal), 10% Total calories: 1,600

Table 10.2   Daily Calorie Intake Based on Body Weight (Body Fat Blitz)

Body weight (lb)	Body weight (kg)	Calories per day	Protein	Carbohydrate	Fat
220	100	2,000	250 g (1,000 cal)	200 g (800 cal)	22 g (200 cal)
200	91	1,800	225 g (900 cal)	180 g (720 cal)	20 g (180 cal)
180	82	1,600	200 g (800 cal)	160 g (640 cal)	18 g (160 cal)
160	73	1,400	175 g (700 cal)	140 g (560 cal)	16 g (140 cal)
140	64	1,200	150 g (600 cal)	120 g (480 cal)	14 g (120 cal)

Nutrient ratio: 50% protein, 40% carbohydrate, 10% fat
Calorie values: 1 g protein = 4 calories; 1 g carbohydrate = 4 calories; 1 g fat = 9 calories
Daily calorie intake = (body weight in pounds × 10) − 10% *or* (body weight in kg × 22) − 10%

Adjust your protein intake by changing the amount of protein powder added to your midafternoon snack or by changing the number of egg whites at breakfast (one egg white contains 6 grams of protein). Similarly, by adjusting the portions of pasta or rice at lunch and dinner, you can increase or decrease your intake of carbohydrate. But remember that the nutrition values in the sample meal plan are only approximate. I strongly recommend that you check nutrition labels on the products you eat because values vary among brands. Supplementing your diet with a fat burner (see chapter 13) may also help promote fat loss.

Progress Measurements

You'll be recording data in two categories: shape and function. In the shape category, record body weight using a scale; measure waist circumference with a tape measure. You can also measure your body fat percentage using a skinfold caliper. Follow the manufacturer's instructions, and record the skin thickness at three sites on your body (typically, the upper arm, waist, and thigh). Calculate the average reading by adding all three measurements and then dividing by 3. The average body fat percentage for males is 15 percent, but a sleek six-pack of abs will show only if your body fat is below 10 percent. As you lose body weight, remember to reduce your calorie intake accordingly to continue making progress.

In the function category, evaluate your fitness during an aerobic exercise of your choice, such as cycling or jogging. Monitor how long you can sustain your heart rate at 70 percent of the maximum. Calculate your target heart rate by subtracting your age from 220 and then multiplying by .7. A person of average fitness should be able to sustain 70 percent of maximum heart rate for 20 minutes. Each week, aim to increase your cardio time by 10 minutes or increase your target heart rate by 5 percent (but no higher than 85% of your maximum heart rate). The harder you work for 30 minutes, the more calories you'll burn. The more calories burned, the greater the fat loss. You can also measure muscle strength by recording the maximum weight you can lift during the last set of each exercise. The stronger the muscle becomes, the bigger it grows. The larger your muscle mass, the more fat you'll burn. Aim to increase the weight on each exercise by 5 percent every two weeks.

Results

After six weeks on this program, you should lose four to six pounds (1.8-2.7 kg) of body fat—about a pound (.5 kg) a week. During this time you'll slice an inch (2.5 cm) off your waist circumference and record a 5 percent drop in body fat.

BODY FAT BLITZ EXERCISE PROGRAM

Routine: Upper–lower two-way split
Cycle: Four days per week
Schedule: Monday, Tuesday, Thursday, Friday
Goal: Lose body fat
Detail: 3 sets of 15, 12, 10 reps
Rest interval: 30 to 60 sec
Workout time: 40 min

Upper body Monday	
Chest	Cable crossover
	Incline dumbbell press
Shoulders	Seated dumbbell lateral raise
	Dumbbell shoulder press
Back	Wide-grip pull-down
	Seated cable row
Arms	Dumbbell curl
	Triceps push-down

Cardio and abs Tuesday	
Cardio	Cycling (30 min)
Abs	Twisting sit-up
	Vertical leg raise

Lower body Thursday	
Quadriceps	Unilateral leg extension
	Machine squat
Hamstrings	Unilateral leg curl
Calves	Donkey calf raise

Cardio and abs Friday	
Cardio	Treadmill (30 min), walking or jogging
Abs	Floor crunch
	Dumbbell pullover

CHEST

Cable Crossover

This is a great isolation exercise for the middle and lower portions of the chest muscle. The maneuver should resemble a bear hug. Stand in the center of the cable crossover machine. With palms turned down, grasp the handles attached to the cables coming from the high pulleys (figure 10.1*a*). Place your feet firmly on the ground about shoulder-width apart. From this crucifix-like position, squeeze the handles down simultaneously in front of your body until your hands meet at hip level (figure 10.1*b*). Hold the contracted position for one second, tightening your chest muscles. Your torso should be tilted forward slightly at the waist. Keep your elbows bent slightly throughout the movement. Slowly return to the start position. Keep your palms turned down, and feel your chest muscles stretch. Hold at the start position for one second and then repeat.

▶ **CHECK IT!** Tilt your torso forward about 25 degrees in relation to the floor. Keep elbows slightly bent with palms turned down. To keep tension on your chest muscles and avoid unwanted stress on your shoulder joints, do not allow your hands to travel above shoulder level.

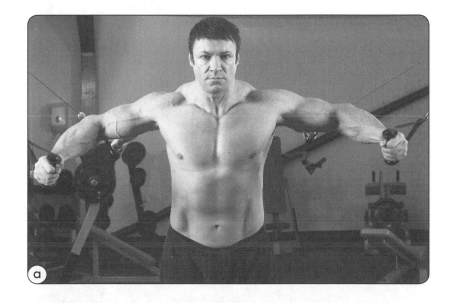

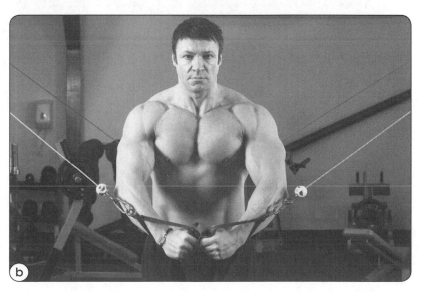

Figure 10.1 Cable crossover: (*a*) Grab the cable handles; (*b*) bring hands in front of your body.

CHEST

Incline Dumbbell Press

Position an adjustable incline bench at a 30- to 45-degree angle. Sit on the bench, grab a dumbbell in each hand, and rest one on each thigh. As you lean back onto the bench, position the dumbbells alongside your chest, palms turned forward (figure 10.2a). Position your feet firmly on the floor for stability. From the start position, press the weights vertically upward over your upper chest (figure 10.2b). Bring the dumbbells together as you raise them. Squeeze your upper chest muscles for one second at the top position, elbows straight. Bending your elbows, lower the weights slowly back to the start position. Hold the dumbbells level with your chest momentarily and then repeat. Inhale on the way down; exhale as you push up. The path the dumbbells travel should be perpendicular to the floor, not to your body.

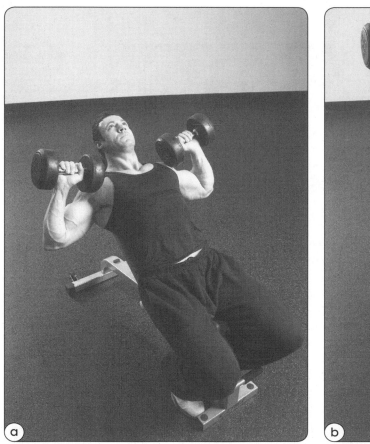 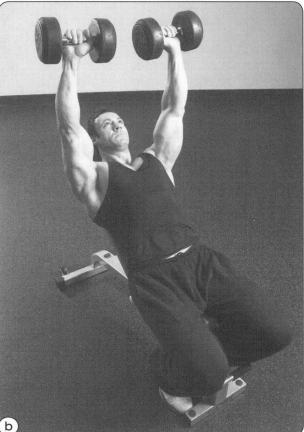

Figure 10.2 Incline dumbbell press: *(a)* Get into position on an incline bench; *(b)* press the weights over your chest.

▶ **CHECK IT!** Do not set the bench at a steep angle, or you'll work your shoulders more than your upper chest.

You can also do the incline bench press using a barbell or a machine. A dumbbell chest press can be performed flat or on an inclined or declined bench.

SHOULDERS

Seated Dumbbell Lateral Raise

Sit upright on the edge of a flat exercise bench. Hold a dumbbell in each hand at arms' length, hanging down by your sides with palms turned in (figure 10.3a). Raise the dumbbells up and out to the sides until they're level with your chin (figure 10.3b). Keep your palms turned down during the lift. Your arms should be slightly bent but elbows kept stiff during the movement. When your elbows reach shoulder level, hold the position momentarily, then lower the weight in a slow, controlled fashion back to the start position. Keep your torso upright during the movement. A slight forward tilt is okay, but don't lean backward.

▶ **CHECK IT!** Do not raise the dumbbells too high because this places undue stress on the shoulder joint. Your hands should be level with your chin, with elbows just about shoulder height. There should be no movement at the elbow joint.

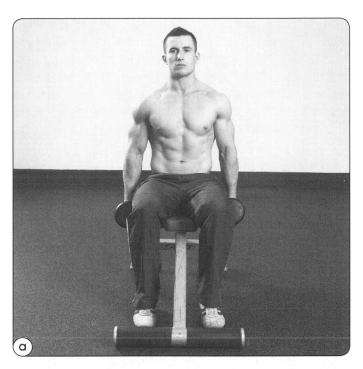

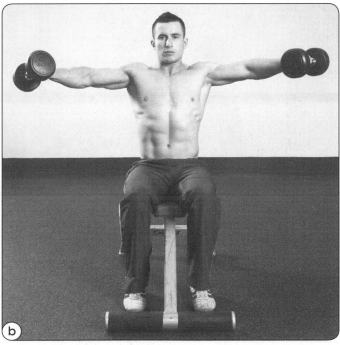

Figure 10.3 Seated dumbbell lateral raise: *(a)* Hold dumbbells at your sides; *(b)* raise the weights.

Dumbbell Shoulder Press

Sit on a bench with the backrest upright at a vertical angle. If the backrest is adjustable, tilt it back 15 to 20 degrees to optimize body position. Hold a dumbbell in each hand, palms turned forward, and lift to shoulder level. Your elbows should point out to the sides. Firmly position your feet on the floor, and lean back onto the bench (figure 10.4a). Press the dumbbells up until your elbows are extended fully overhead (figure 10.4b). Pause momentarily, contracting your deltoid muscles. Slowly lower the weights to shoulder level. Pause for one second and then repeat. You may also perform this exercise on a seated front press machine.

▶ **CHECK IT!** Do not allow the dumbbells to stray back and forth during the movement. The weights should move in one plane, vertically up and down, perpendicular to the floor.

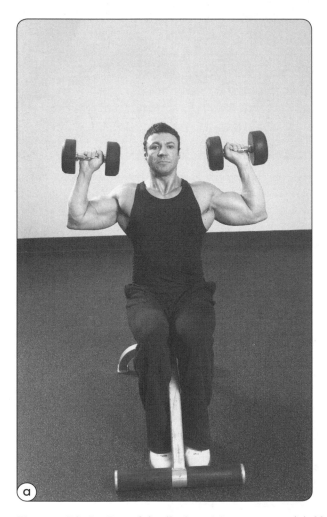 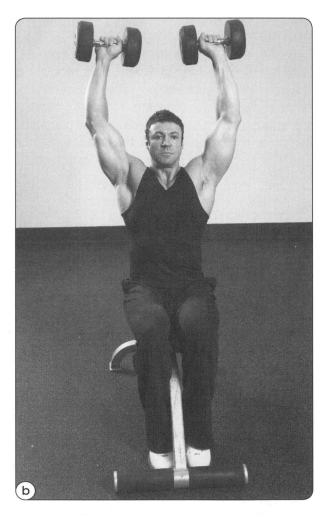

Figure 10.4 Dumbbell shoulder press: *(a)* Hold dumbbells at shoulder level; *(b)* press the dumbbells overhead.

Wide-Grip Pull-Down

Sit at a cable pull-down machine, facing inward, and position your thighs under the pads. Grasp the bar in an overhand grip, palms turned forward, with hands about six inches (15 cm) wider than shoulder width. From the start position, with arms fully extended overhead, lean your torso back about 30 degrees from the vertical plane (figure 10.5*a*). Begin the repetition by pulling the bar down toward the top of your chest (figure 10.5*b*). Think of your hands as hooks. Make your upper back muscles do the work, pulling your elbows down and back. Hold the bar above your collarbone for one second, contracting the latissimus muscles. Slowly return to the start position. This exercise develops width in your back muscles.

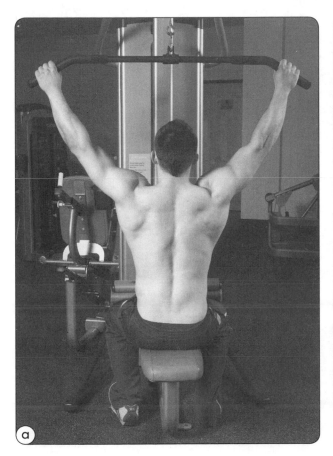 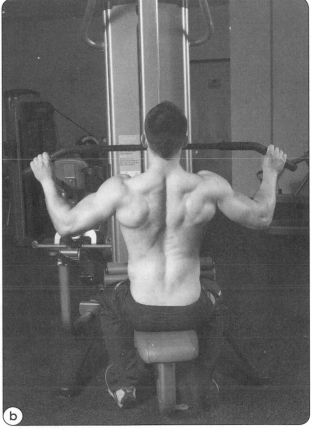

Figure 10.5 Wide-grip pull-down: *(a)* Extend arms overhead; *(b)* bring the bar toward your chest.

▶ **CHECK IT!** Do not pull the bar down below your collarbones. Do not lean back too far or pull the weight down using momentum.

You can also do pull-downs using a reverse underhand grip on the bar with palms turned toward you, as described in chapter 14. If you don't have access to a pull-down machine, the same movement can be done using a chin-up bar (chapter 7).

Seated Cable Row

Position yourself at a seated row station. Grab the handlebar attached to the low pulley cable with your arms extended in front of you. Place your feet shoulder-width apart on the footplate. Sit up straight and pull your shoulders back (figure 10.6*a*). From the start position, pull the handlebar to your upper abdomen, moving your elbows backward as far as you can. Hold the contracted position momentarily, squeezing your back muscles (figure 10.6*b*). Don't lean backward. Keeping your spine straight, slowly return to the start position and then repeat. This is a great exercise to build thickness and strength in the middle and lower sections of your back. You can perform the seated cable row using a variety of grips. The handlebar attachment affords a narrow vertical grip with palms facing one another. Attaching a straight bar to the low cable allows you to use a wider hand placement with an under- or overhand grip. My personal preference is the handlebar grip.

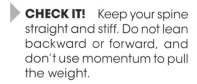 **CHECK IT!** Keep your spine straight and stiff. Do not lean backward or forward, and don't use momentum to pull the weight.

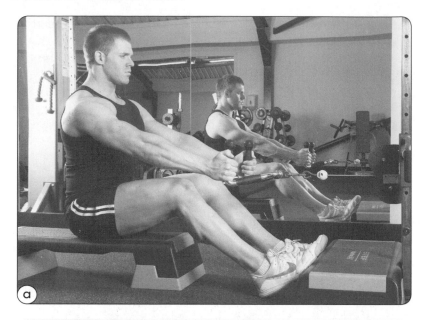

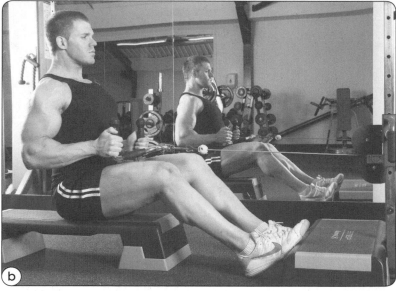

Figure 10.6 Seated cable row: *(a)* Hold the handlebar with arms extended; *(b)* pull back toward your abdomen.

Dumbbell Curl

Grab a pair of dumbbells, and sit on the edge of a bench. Start with your arms straight at your sides (figure 10.7a). Do this exercise with one arm at a time—the right arm curls first, then the left arm, and so on. With palms turned forward, bend the right elbow, lifting the dumbbell toward your right shoulder (figure 10.7b). Keep your upper arm and torso still; let your biceps do the work. When the dumbbell reaches shoulder level, pause for one second before lowering the weight slowly. When the dumbbell returns to the start position, pause while you perform the next repetition using the left arm. Alternate reps between the right and left arms until the set is complete.

▶ **CHECK IT!** To maximize biceps contraction, turn your palms to face upward as you raise the weight.

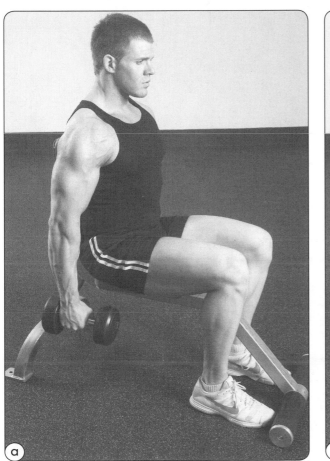
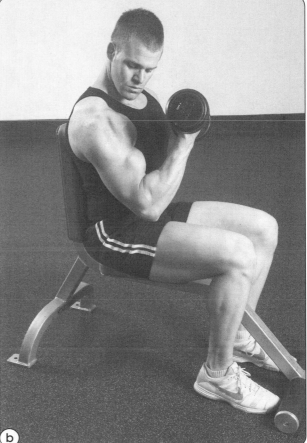

Figure 10.7 Dumbbell curl: *(a)* Sit on a bench, arms at your sides; *(b)* curl weight toward your shoulder.

Triceps Push-Down

Attach a short bar to the cable of a high pulley. Grip the bar with hands slightly closer than shoulder-width apart and palms turned down. Position your upper arms perpendicular to the ground, keeping the elbows in at your sides. In the start position, the bar is at nipple level and elbows are bent past 90 degrees (figure 10.8a). Push the bar down toward your thighs until your arms are straight and your elbows lock (figure 10.8b). Keep the upper arms close to your body. Flex your triceps at the bottom position for one count. Slowly return to the start position, hold momentarily, and repeat.

▶ **CHECK IT!**   Keep your upper arms stiff; motion should occur only at the elbows.

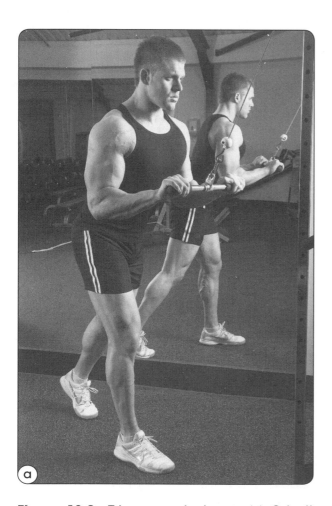 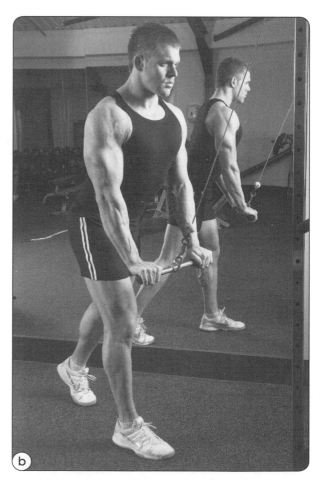

Figure 10.8 Triceps push-down: (a) Grip the bar on the cable machine; (b) push the bar toward your thighs.

Cardio and Abs (Tuesday)

CARDIO

Spend 30 minutes on a stationary bike, keeping your heart rate in the target range (see page 84 for calculation).

ABS

Twisting Sit-Up

This exercise is a variation of the decline sit-up described in chapter 7. The movement incorporates a slight twist of your torso to work the serratus and oblique muscles. The decline bench should be at a 20-degree head-down angle to the floor. Position your feet under the roller pad with the backs of your knees on the knee pad. Lie back and place your hands behind your head (figure 10.9a). As you crunch up from the bottom position, direct your right elbow toward your left knee (figure 10.9b). Feel the contraction in your right oblique muscles. Hold for one second, then return to the start position. During the second repetition, direct your left elbow to your right knee to work your left oblique muscles. Repeat, alternating between left and right sides. As you gain strength, increase the number of reps, or tilt the bench at a steeper angle.

▶ **CHECK IT!** Do not lean back too far; this releases tension from the abdominals and places unnecessary stress on the lower back.

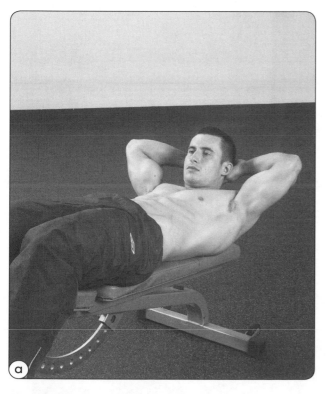 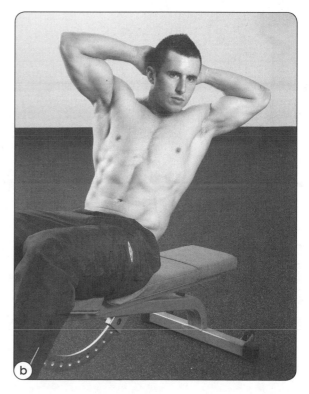

Figure 10. 9 Twisting sit-up: (a) Lie back with hands behind head; (b) curl up, directing right elbow toward left knee.

Vertical Leg Raise

Hanging vertical from a chin-up bar, support your weight with your hands at arms' length. Your legs should be hanging straight down, feet side by side (figure 10.10*a*). From the start position, raise your legs at the hips while bending your knees. Pull your thighs up toward your chest, keeping your legs together (figure 10.10*b*). Hold the top position momentarily, contracting your abs. Then slowly lower your legs down to the start position and repeat. This is a terrific exercise for your lower abs.

▶ **CHECK IT!**   Lower your legs down slowly to keep tension on your abs. Avoid swinging your legs.

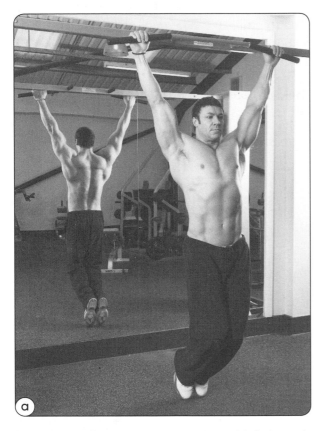 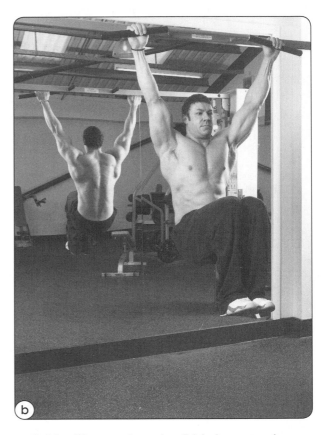

Figure 10.10   Vertical leg raise: *(a)* Support your weight with your hands; *(b)* bring your knees toward your chest.

Lower Body (Thursday)

QUADRICEPS

Unilateral Leg Extension

Sit at a leg extension machine. Adjust the backrest so the back of your knee fits snugly against the seat and your whole thigh is supported. Position your ankle under the roller pad. If the pad is adjustable, position it so it rests just above your ankle on the lowest part of your shin. Grip the handles on the side of the machine for support (figure 10.11a). Using one leg at a time, contract the quadriceps to straighten one knee, while the other leg remains stationary (figure 10.11b). Lift the weight all the way up until your knee is straight. Pause for one second at the top, flexing the quadriceps muscle. Slowly lower the weight until your knee bends to 90 degrees. Hold the weight momentarily in the bottom position and repeat. Upon completion of the set number of reps, let the fatigued leg hang down, and do the exercise with the other leg.

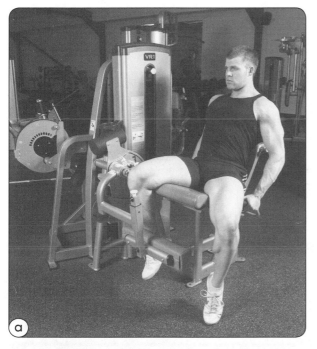 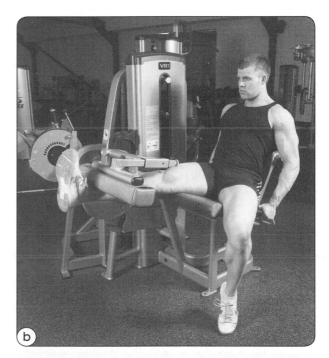

Figure 10.11 Unilateral leg extension: *(a)* Sit in the leg extension machine; *(b)* straighten one leg at a time.

You can also do this exercise in the standard fashion using both legs at once, as described in chapter 7. The advantage of the unilateral version is that it requires extra effort and burns more calories.

▶ **CHECK IT!** Do not bend your knee beyond 90 degrees, as this will inflict unnecessary stress across the knee joint.

Machine Squat

Use a Smith machine if one is available. Position the bar of the machine centrally across the upper portion of your back. Stand with your feet shoulder-width apart, slightly in front of the plane of your body, with toes pointing forward (figure 10.12*a*). This is the start position. Begin the repetition by bending your knees and slowly lowering your hips straight down until your thighs are parallel to the floor (figure 10.12*b*). During the movement, be sure to keep your back straight, chin up, and head looking forward. Once you reach the bottom position, push the weight up using your thighs and hips until your knees are straight. On a Smith machine, the movement occurs in a single plane, vertically up and down, perpendicular to the floor. Inhale deeply during the descent, and exhale on the way up.

▶ **CHECK IT!** To reduce the chance of knee injury, avoid squatting below parallel. Position your feet about six inches (15 cm) in front of the plane of your body during machine squats to optimize trajectory.

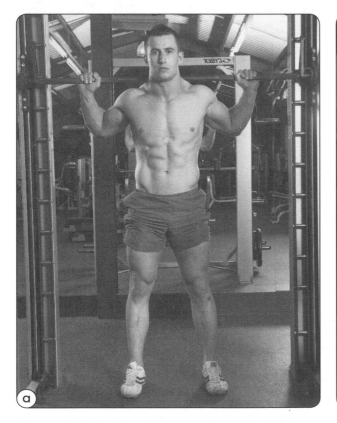 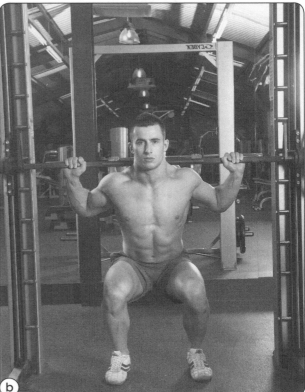

Figure 10.12 Machine squat: *(a)* Get into position in the machine; *(b)* lower the weight by bending your knees.

Unilateral Leg Curl

Position on the leg curl machine, and place one ankle on the roller pad, leaving your other leg to hang free (figure 10.13*a*). Grip the handles to stabilize your body. From the start position, curl the weight up by bending your knee (figure 10.13*b*). Hold the contracted position for one second. Slowly return the weight to the start position with your leg almost straight. Hold momentarily and then repeat. After you've completed the set number of reps with one leg, do the same for the opposite leg.

▶ **CHECK IT!** Do not hyperextend your leg at the bottom, as this will remove tension from the hamstrings as well as place unwanted stress through your knee joint.

Unilateral leg curls can be performed (one leg at a time) on the *lying* leg curl machine, or alternatively using a *standing* leg curl machine.

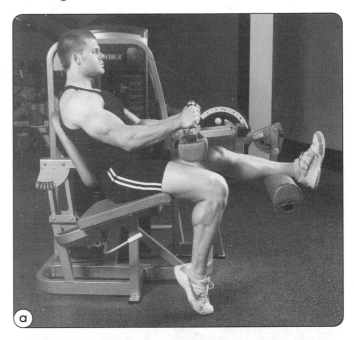

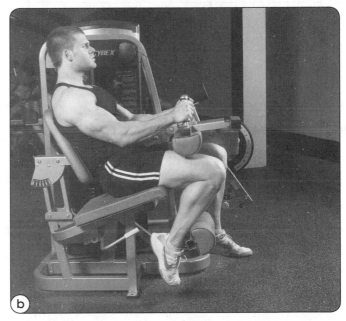

Figure 10.13 Unilateral leg curl: *(a)* Sit in the leg curl machine; *(b)* bring heel toward buttock.

Donkey Calf Raise

Place a calf block or a three-inch (8 cm) block of wood in front of an exercise bench. Position the balls of your feet on the block, bend forward at the hips, and support your upper body on the bench. Have your training partner sit astride your hips so that his body weight is directly above your calf muscles. Keeping your knees locked, lower your heels, stretching out your calf muscles (figure 10.14a). From the start position, raise your heels as high as you can, lifting your partner's weight vertically upward. At the top position, squeeze your calf muscles and hold for one count (figure 10.14b). Slowly lower your heels back to the start position. Hold the stretch momentarily and then repeat.

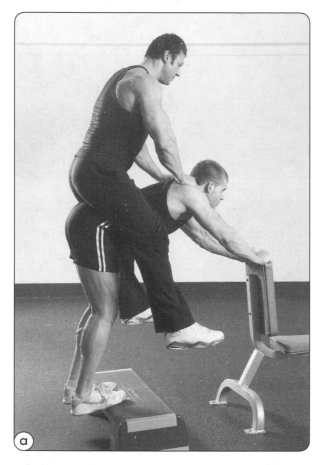
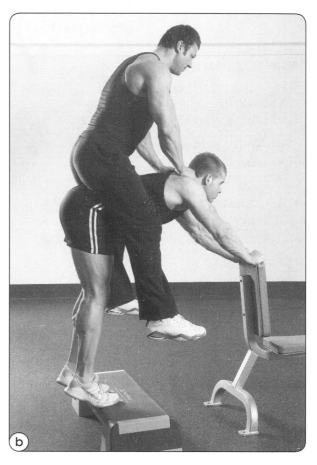

Figure 10.14 Donkey calf raise: *(a)* Get into position on the calf block; *(b)* raise your heels upward.

▶ **CHECK IT!** Keep your back straight, and keep your knees stiff but slightly bent.

You can also do the straight-leg donkey calf raise on a calf machine where the weight is transmitted through a pad that rests across your lower back. If you don't have a training partner or access to this type of calf machine, do standing calf raises, as described in chapter 7.

CARDIO

Spend 30 minutes on a treadmill, keeping your heart rate within target range (see page 84 for calculation). Walk briskly or jog, depending on your level of fitness.

ABS

Floor Crunch

Lie on the floor with your hands behind your head. Place your feet flat on the floor about a foot (30 cm) from your buttocks (figure 10.15a). Begin the exercise by pushing your lower back into the floor. Roll your shoulders up, keeping your knees and hips still (figure 10.15b). Crunch your chest forward until your abs are fully contracted. Your shoulders will raise only a few inches off the floor. Keep your lower spine in contact with the floor. Hold the contracted position for one second, lower your shoulders, and then repeat. This exercise works the upper portion of your abdominals. You can also do this exercise on an abdominal crunch machine (page 185).

▶ **CHECK IT!** Avoid bending your head too far forward, as this will place unnecessary stress on your neck.

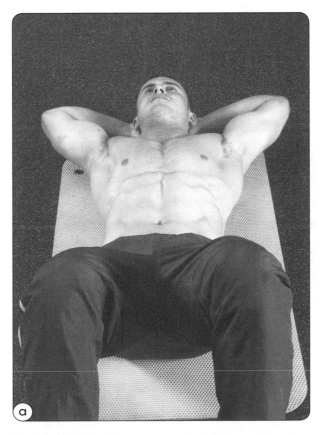 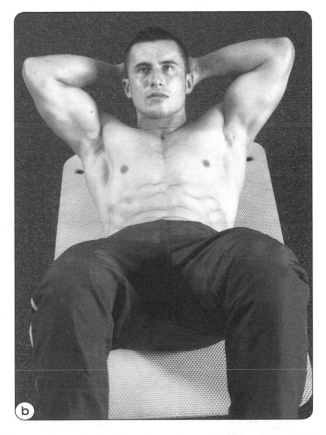

Figure 10.15 Floor crunch: *(a)* Lie on the floor with your hands behind your head; *(b)* raise your shoulders off the floor.

Dumbbell Pullover

This is not a typical abdominal exercise, but it does develop the fingerlike serratus muscles that fan out from the armpits into the upper abs. The exercise helps expand the rib cage and feels therapeutic when you're out of breath immediately after a cardio session. Lie supine across a flat exercise bench with only your upper back resting on the bench. Position your feet firmly on the floor to stabilize your lower torso. Grab a dumbbell by placing your palms against the inside of the plates at one end, positioning your hands together so that your index fingers and thumbs form a diamond shape. Extend your arms straight up above your head so that the dumbbell hangs directly over your face (figure 10.16a). From this start position, lower the dumbbell backward until your hands pass just below the level of your head (figure 10.16b). Your arms should bend slightly during the movement. Inhale deeply as you lower the weight and achieve a full stretch on the rib cage. Pull the weight back to the start position, following the same wide arc, exhaling as you do so. You can also perform this movement using a pullover machine.

▶ **CHECK IT!** Deep breathing is essential during this exercise. Do not let your arms drop too far behind your head because this risks shoulder injury.

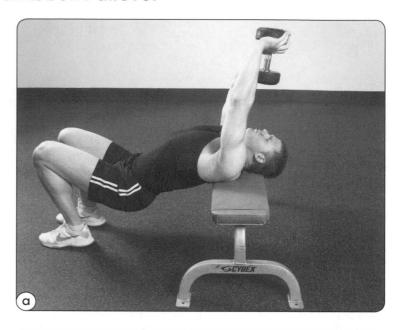

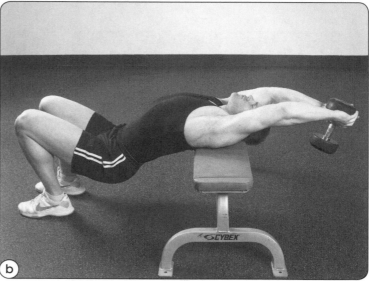

Figure 10.16 Dumbbell pullover: *(a)* Hold the dumbbell over your face; *(b)* lower the dumbbell.

Chiseling the Ultimate Body

Part IV gives you the advanced tools you need for chiseling the ultimate body. I'll teach you how to integrate your workouts and your diet for maximum benefit—the secret combination that makes the magic. Climb the 12 steps up the ladder of intensity in chapter 11 to discover how to turn up the heat at the gym. Train beyond pain and enter the zone of hyperintensity, pushing your muscles past the point of failure to generate extreme muscular development. What about anabolic steroids? Look no further. The real deal is revealed in chapter 12—the good, the bad, and the ugly truth about these muscle-building drugs. Are there safer ways to fuel your intensified workouts? You bet. I've put together a super supplement stack for surefire results in chapter 13. Find out which nutritional aids work and how to use them effectively. The hybrid hard body program in chapter 14 is my personal formula for the ultimate physique. This program is an advanced system designed to build, shape, and sculpt your torso by maximizing muscle growth and fat loss at the same time.

Climbing the Ladder of Intensity

Body sculpting has two extremes. At one end, the goal is generating muscle mass. At the other, the focus is fat loss. The middle ground is a combination of the two—a hybrid system. This is a more advanced program that requires a refinement of training techniques to raise the intensity of your workouts.

Before revealing the tricks to turbocharging your workout, let's clarify what intensity actually means. Intensity is the degree of effort, or the percentage of momentary ability. At the point of muscular failure, 100 percent intensity (effort) is required to complete the last rep. The muscle is pushed to its limit and must contract to its maximum capability to complete the task. Exhausted and disrupted by this demanding stimulus, muscle fibers grow in size.

The question is, can you be sure that all muscle fibers have been recruited and exhausted at the point of failure during that last rep? The answer is probably not. So, is it possible to generate even more intensity and stimulate the muscle further? The answer is yes. You must go beyond failure and step into the zone of higher intensity to ensure that every last muscle fiber is maximally stimulated to the point of exhaustion. The rule of high-intensity training is that the set is just beginning when the muscle fails. To climb the ladder of intensity, your training techniques must evolve in a positive direction by shifting up a gear to a higher level. There are several ways in which workout intensity can evolve. These methods require manipulating the core elements of your exercise program, namely the resistance, the sets, the rest intervals, the exercise combinations, and the repetition itself. Here are the techniques for intensifying your training.

12 STEPS TO INTENSIFY

The 12 steps up the ladder of intensity are as follows:

1. Increase resistance.
2. Add an exercise.

3. Shorten rest intervals.
4. Prefatigue the muscle.
5. Add supersets.
6. Add drop sets.
7. Change repetition tempo.
8. Use power-paused repetitions.
9. Use partial repetitions.
10. Use static contraction.
11. Add negative reps.
12. Add forced reps.

Step 1: Increase resistance   Gradually increasing the weight you lift intensifies the stimulus the muscle receives at the point of failure during the last repetition. So if you add an extra 10 pounds (4.5 kg) to your six-rep maximum, your muscles receive a greater stimulus than they did during the previous workout. Added resistance raises the intensity, and the muscle will go beyond its previous point of failure. A larger stimulus provides a bigger challenge for your muscles. As they get stronger, they get bigger. This is the basic theory behind progressive resistance training—as you get stronger, you add more resistance.

Aim to add more resistance to each exercise every two to four weeks. A word of caution, however. Your maximum weight is that which you can lift for 6 repetitions while using perfect form. Performing fewer than 6 reps of your maximum weight and then trying to add resistance carries a high risk of injury. Only when you're capable of performing 8 to 10 reps on your previous best weight can you safely increase the resistance by 5 percent and try for 6 reps on the new weight.

Step 2: Add an exercise   Larger muscle groups such as the chest, shoulders, and back benefit from several exercises that target different portions of the muscle. Working the muscle from a different angle intensifies the overall stimulus by bringing additional muscle fibers into action. For instance, a set of flat bench presses performed to failure does not necessarily exhaust the muscle fibers of the upper chest. Add an incline exercise to maximally stimulate the upper (clavicular) portion of the muscle. Similarly, shoulder presses recruit and exhaust the front deltoids, but the lateral (side) and rear heads of the muscle remain relatively underworked. For complete muscular development, all the muscle fibers must be recruited and exhausted in every section of the muscle. Adding additional exercises is a way to ensure maximum intensity for all portions of the muscle. But remember—new movements are required only if you're targeting a separate portion of the muscle. There is little benefit in adding an identical exercise.

Step 3: Shorten rest intervals   The less time you rest between sets and exercises, the more intense the workout becomes. Shortening rest intervals is a safe, effective way to raise intensity. The muscle fibers exhausted by the first set don't have time to recover, so during the second set the muscle must recruit even more fibers to move the resistance. Shortening the interval between sets also burns more calories—a great way to build muscle and burn fat at the same time.

Step 4: Prefatigue the muscle   This technique relates to exercise sequence. It employs an isolation exercise to prefatigue a muscle before moving to a compound movement. The goal is to recruit and exhaust more muscle fibers, thereby generating a more effective growth response. Performing an isolation exercise exhausts the target muscle so that when you proceed to the compound exercise, the fatigued primary muscle will fail before the smaller assistance muscles. For example, perform chest flys to prefatigue the pectorals before performing bench presses. This ensures that the chest muscles fail before the weaker triceps muscles that assist in the pressing movement. You don't want to have to terminate your set of bench presses because the triceps have reached the point of failure before the pectorals. Similarly, preexhausting the deltoid with lateral raises makes the deltoid work harder during shoulder presses, sparing the weaker triceps muscles. I recommend the prefatigue technique as standard practice in my training programs, so you should already be using it to good effect.

Step 5: Add supersets   A superset involves performing two exercises back to back without a rest interval. Essentially, this technique takes the prefatigue concept to a higher level of intensity. The difference is that you don't give the muscle time to rest between two exercises. By proceeding immediately to the second set, additional muscle fibers are forced to work after the other fibers have already failed. The second set raises intensity by taking the muscle beyond failure. When you superset two exercises for the same muscle group, the total time under tension increases, and you tap into different muscle fibers as you go from one exercise to the other. This activates a greater percentage of the muscle area, which stimulates extra growth. Examples of superset combinations include leg extensions followed by squats; leg curls followed by stiff-leg deadlifts; chest flys followed by bench presses; deltoid raises followed by shoulder presses; and lat pull-downs followed by rows. If you combine more than two exercises in this way without a rest interval, the sequence becomes a giant set.

Step 6: Add drop sets   A drop set is a method of extending an exercise beyond failure by reducing the weight so that you can perform more reps. When you reach muscular failure at the end of a set, immediately decrease the resistance by 25 to 40 percent and continue the exercise, squeezing out a few more reps until you reach failure with the lowered weight. Rest only for the few seconds it takes to reduce the weight. Drop sets are performed easily on machines where all you need to do is reposition the weight pin to a lower level. During barbell exercises, the plates must be stripped from the bar. For added intensity, do several successive drop sets (double-drop or triple-drop sets) by continuing to reduce the weight each time you reach momentary muscular failure. You can also do drop sets with dumbbells using the down-the-rack technique. Each time the muscle fails, use progressively lighter dumbbells nonstop until the muscles are completely fatigued. This is an excellent method of annihilating the deltoids with dumbbell lateral raises. Let's say your work set fails on the eighth rep with 30-pound (13.5 kg) dumbbells. Proceed immediately down the rack to the 20-pound (9 kg) dumbbells, and continue the exercise to failure again. Then drop to the 10-pound (4.5 kg) dumbbells (and so on), continuing the movement until the muscle fails again. By the time you've worked all the way down the rack, it will feel as if someone is blowtorching your deltoids!

Step 7: Change repetition tempo   The speed at which you perform a repetition affects intensity. A repetition performed at a fast tempo typically allows the use of a heavier weight, but the rapid acceleration introduces momentum.

Excessive momentum with quick repetitions decreases muscle effort. Performing a repetition slowly reduces momentum and maximizes muscle tension throughout the range of motion. Remember that it's the weight (or tension) on the muscle that counts, not the weight on the barbell. Slowing down rep tempo is a method of increasing intensity. This doesn't mean you should use slow-motion reps all the time. On the contrary, varying the rep tempo is the best way to go. Switching from a slow tempo (two seconds down, two seconds up) to a fast tempo (one second down, one second up) taps into different muscle fibers, ensuring maximum muscle recruitment. This effect is also influenced by changing the relative speed of the positive and negative phases of the rep. Slowing the positive phase accentuates the concentric contraction (e.g., two seconds down, four seconds up), whereas doing the negative phase slowly focuses on the eccentric contraction (e.g., four seconds down, two seconds up). To continue adding muscle mass and generating new levels of intensity, the concept of varying rep tempo is very important.

Step 8: Use power-paused repetitions A paused rep allows you to push past the point of positive muscular failure by providing your muscle with a few seconds' rest in static isometric contraction mode. When you reach muscular failure at the end of a set, hold the weight still for a few seconds. The power pause can be taken at any point during the positive phase of the repetition. Having taken advantage of a few valuable seconds of rest, you'll be able to perform one more complete repetition past the point of failure. Using the paused rep, the set is extended beyond failure in a stop-and-go fashion.

Step 9: Use partial repetitions By definition, the point of muscular failure occurs when you're no longer able to complete the last repetition through the full range of motion. However, despite not being able to complete a full repetition, the muscle can still perform a partial repetition that employs only a portion of the lift. That shorter arc of motion might involve any part of the repetition—the beginning, midpoint, or end phase. Usually, the partial rep is performed within the range where the muscle is stronger. For instance, a partial rep during a bench press involves the first phase of the lift as the bar is pushed up off the chest. This is the portion where the pectorals generate the most power. Similarly, during shoulder presses, the focus is on the deltoid during the initial phase. With all pressing movements, the triceps do most of the work as your arms approach the lockout position. Instead of quitting when you can no longer complete a full repetition, do partial reps to take the muscle beyond the point of positive failure.

Step 10: Use static contraction A static, or isometric, contraction is the force generated in a muscle when there's no motion and the weight is held still. Because an isometric contraction is stronger than a concentric contraction, it is a means of continuing the set beyond the point of concentric muscular failure. Even though you can no longer lift the weight, your muscle is able to hold the weight static. By squeezing a peak static contraction in the muscle, the muscle is forced to continue working past the point of failure. Hold the weight as long as you can until you reach the point of isometric muscular failure. When the weight finally overcomes the isometric strength, your muscle will be ready to burst.

Step 11: Add negative reps The strongest phase of a repetition is the negative phase of lowering the weight. Even though the muscle has failed during the positive phase and fatigued during a static contraction, the more powerful eccentric contraction is still able to control the weight as it is lowered. This high-intensity technique uses the strong eccentric (or negative) muscle contraction to perform extra work beyond concentric and isometric muscular failure. The negative rep is performed by lowering the weight down as s-l-o-w-l-y as possible, resisting the pull of gravity. To perform additional negative reps, ask your training partner to lift the weight back up to the top position.

Step 12: Add forced reps   A forced rep is an assisted repetition. When you reach the point of positive muscular failure, your training partner helps you perform another complete repetition by assisting with the lift. Your partner provides just enough help for you to complete another positive-phase repetition. This technique allows you to push past the point of positive failure. You'll need an experienced partner to fine-tune the resistance, taking just enough pressure off the bar so that you're forced to work as hard as possible to squeeze out a few extra complete reps.

HYPERINTENSITY TRAINING

Climbing the ladder is an apt phrase for stepping up intensity. To go beyond failure, you can take one step at a time or jump several steps together. It requires 100 percent effort to complete the last repetition to the point of momentary muscular failure. Taking one step up the ladder goes beyond failure, forcing the muscle to recruit extra fibers to generate higher intensity. Jumping several steps up the ladder at once goes beyond the pain to inflict absolute, complete muscular failure, generating hyperintensity.

How does this technique work? Well, let's say you're squeezing out that last rep and you've reached the point of failure. By employing one of the 12 techniques, such as a drop set or some forced reps, you'll go beyond failure into the realm of high intensity. However, if you use several of these advanced techniques together in sequence, such as a static contraction, a negative rep, and a forced rep, you can train past failure over and over again. This brutal multistep system pushes your muscle beyond the pain into the zone of hyperintensity. You've manipulated that final repetition and extended the last set by jumping several steps up the ladder of intensity. Hyperintensity is hard core. It takes your muscles beyond failure and then some. Your muscles will burn and scream with pain. Give them no mercy. In response to the onslaught of hyperintensity, they'll have no choice but to grow.

So, do you need to use all 12 steps to generate intense workouts? Not necessarily. But the more tricks you have in your gym bag, the more versatile your workouts can become. High-demand techniques such as forced reps and negative reps require the assistance of an experienced training partner. Most of the other methods, such as drop sets and partial reps, can be performed without a spotter, so you can venture into the zone of hyperintensity all by yourself. It's worth mentioning that turning up the intensity is easier (and safer) using machines and dumbbells rather than barbells. If you fail to complete the last rep on most machines, you're safe with or without help.

EXTREME TRAINING

Let's look at some examples to illustrate how to incorporate the brutal tactics of hyperintensity into your workouts. (Just when you thought it was safe to go to the gym!)

Deltoid Demolition

Before you start, warm up your shoulders with a set or two of lateral raises, using a pair of light dumbbells. The first exercise is the dumbbell lateral raise (see page 69). Line up three sets of dumbbells in order of descending weight on the rack, beginning with your eight-repetition-maximum weight. For example, if your eight-repetition-maximum weight is a pair of 30-pound (13.5 kg) dumbbells, place a pair of 20-pound (9 kg) dumbbells next in line, then a pair of 15-pound (7 kg) dumbbells. Grab the heaviest pair of dumbbells, and begin doing dumbbell lateral raises in a steady manner (one second up, one second down). When you fail on the eighth rep, hold the dumbbells in a static contraction at the top for as long as you can. Then slowly perform a negative rep, lowering the dumbbells to your sides. Place them back on the rack and immediately grab the next set of dumbbells. Without resting, continue the exercise until you reach failure a second time, hold the static contraction then slowly lower the weights back down. Switch dumbbells again, picking up the lightest pair, and resume the exercise. Squeeze those reps out until you reach failure for a third time. Despite the screaming pain in your delts, hold the weight in a static contraction on the last rep for five seconds. Slowly lower the weights to your sides, using a negative rep. Finish with a final blast of partial reps, raising the dumbbells halfway up (about 45 degrees) until you fail for a fourth time.

By this time, your deltoids will be on fire, but you're not done yet. As you catch your breath, head straight for the seated front shoulder press machine. Place the weight pin at your eight-repetition-maximum weight and sit down. No need for a warm-up this time—your shoulders are good to go! Squeeze out six to eight reps on the front press to the point of failure. Slowly lower the weight in a negative fashion for a count of five. Then relocate the weight pin, dropping the resistance by about 30 percent, and continue the exercise until you hit failure again. Hold the weight just short of lockout for a count of five in a static contraction. Finally, lower the weight slowly to perform one last negative repetition.

Phew, that's it! Your deltoids are a done deal in under 10 minutes. All you did was two extended sets involving two exercises, but using a combination of hyperintensity techniques, including preexhaustion, drop sets, static contraction, partial reps, and negative reps, your deltoids have been blasted out of orbit. As a result, you inflicted a massive hypertrophic growth response, guaranteed to give you boulder shoulders.

Biceps Blast

All you need in order to blast your biceps is one extended set of hyperintensity. One of the best exercises to achieve this is the one-arm biceps curl on a preacher bench. The movement can be done using a dumbbell or a machine. With your upper arm supported on the pad, the biceps must do all the work. By using one arm at a time, you don't need a training partner to elicit hyperintensity.

First get your biceps into the groove with a light warm-up set. Select a weight equivalent to your six-rep maximum—one arm, remember. Perform the curls in a slow, controlled manner (two seconds up, two seconds down). Once you start to fail, use your free hand to assist in completing an additional six forced repetitions past your failure point. On that final rep, hold the weight in a static peak contraction without assistance for as long as you can. As the isometric contraction begins to fail, perform a negative rep, slowly lowering the weight. When the weight reaches the bottom, use your free hand to lift the weight back up and perform another three negative reps in the same way. By the time you've completed that last negative, your biceps will be bursting at the seams with a pounding muscle pump.

That's all it takes: one extended set taken beyond failure, using a mind-blowing sequence of forced reps, static contraction, and negatives. If you're feeling really masochistic, you can add a drop set, but don't forget your other arm's turn for torture.

Chiseling the Chest

With just two exercises, you can pulverize your pectorals. You'll need to do an isolation exercise to prefatigue the muscle and then a compound pressing movement. I prefer to start with machine flys, but cable crossovers will also do the trick.

Warm up with one or two light sets before loading the machine with your 8- to 10-rep-maximum weight. Focus your mind on the task ahead; once you start the roller coaster, there's no getting off. Begin the set of flys with slow, precise reps. When you hit failure at 8 to 10 reps, reduce the resistance by 30 to 40 percent, and continue the set without rest. Squeeze out as many reps as you can to failure, then drop the weight again by another 30 to 40 percent. Keep pumping out the reps until you fail a third time, then squeeze your hands together in the fully contracted position until you can no longer sustain the static contraction. Let the weight down slowly using a negative rep for a count of five seconds.

By now, your pectoral muscles will be scorching with pain, but the battle ain't over yet. Take a minute to catch your breath and make your way to the Smith machine for incline bench presses. Load the machine with your eight-rep maximum weight and set the backrest at a 30- to 45-degree incline. Perform slow, rhythmic reps until you hit failure, then get your partner to assist for four forced reps. On the last rep, stop short of lockout and hold that bar in a static contraction, squeezing the pecs for five seconds. Perform a slow negative rep, lowering the weight under control toward your chest. Ask your partner to lift the weight back up, then do three more negative reps.

At this point your chest should be annihilated to the point of extreme exhaustion, but if you want more punishment, reduce the weight by 30 to 40 percent and perform a drop set to failure followed by four to six forced reps. That's your hyperintense chest workout.

INTENSITY RULES

Beyond-failure training requires an extreme effort from an already fatigued muscle. The typical work set is extended and then some. Indeed, when the muscle fails, the set is just beginning. Don't underestimate the exercise-induced assault on your body. Here are a few tips to help you reap the rewards of hyperintensity. Remember: timing, strategy, safety, and recovery.

Timing So when should you add intensity to your workouts? Well, simple steps such as increasing resistance, prefatiguing the muscle, shortening rest intervals, and changing repetition tempo can be incorporated frequently for any muscle during any set on any exercise. However, the more demanding techniques such as drop sets, partials, negatives, or forced repetitions push the muscle beyond failure and are best saved for the *last* set of the *last* exercise for any given muscle group. In other words, you end an exercise and polish off the muscle with high intensity. Clearly, you should not be trying a forced rep during the warm-up set.

Strategy The most demanding techniques are forced reps and negative reps performed using your six- to eight-rep maximum weight. Going beyond failure with the maximum possible weight is the ultimate stimulus for gains in mass and strength. However, these extreme techniques demand a high level of caution. Get assistance from a training partner. Taking your maximum weight past failure with forced reps and negative reps should be used strategically and sparingly. Performing a few forced reps constitutes *one* step beyond failure. If you follow that with some negatives, it's another step. Should you then decide to add a drop set, you climb further up the ladder, and so on. Depending on how many different steps you add beyond failure, you extend the set to higher levels of intensity. But remember, there's a fine line between maximizing muscle stimulus and going one step too far, leading to overtraining or injury.

Safety Going beyond failure is less dangerous when you use machines or dumbbells. It's also safer to do a drop set before you perform forced reps or negative reps. Manipulating the repetition is less hazardous after you've gone to failure on a drop set because the weight has been reduced by 30 to 40 percent. When you climb the ladder of intensity, the risk of injury increases. The well-known bodybuilder's mantra "no pain, no gain" is to an extent true. But the pain you want is a muscular pain, a burning sensation felt deep within the muscle belly that results from muscular fatigue and the buildup of lactic acid inside the tissues. The pain you *don't* want is a sharp, knifelike pain felt in a tendon or joint just before something breaks under excessive strain. Learn to recognize the difference between these two pain sensations. A sharp pain is a warning signal of impending injury—stop the exercise immediately or risk joint or tendon damage.

Sore Muscles:
I ache terribly after a workout. How can I speed up my muscle recovery?

Intense exercise inflicts muscle fiber disruption, causing postworkout pain, spasm, and stiffness. To expedite recovery, try the following suggestions.

1. Static (nonballistic) stretching, before and after your workout, will prevent or alleviate muscle spasm.
2. Soak in a hot bath; heat helps muscles relax.
3. Rest. Muscles need rest to repair the damage inflicted by an intense workout, and your body will perform better when you get adequate sleep.
4. Replenish your muscles with a postworkout protein and carbohydrate drink. Glutamine supplementation also aids recovery.

Recovery   The hyperintensity experience is not your typical day at the gym. It's the ultimate challenge, an annihilation of the muscle. As such, this exercise-induced insult requires seven days to repair. If you want to grow from these techniques, you must allow adequate rest for that tortured muscle group to recover between workouts.

Having discovered the 12 steps up the ladder of intensity, you now know how to turn up the heat at the gym, pushing your muscles past the point of failure to maximize muscular development. In the next chapter we discuss anabolic steroids—the good, the bad, and the ugly *truth* about these muscle-building drugs.

Anabolic Overdrive

In the quest for size and strength, many people turn to the dark side of the force, selling their souls to the devil in exchange for an extra inch on their biceps or another plate on their bench press. An estimated one in every five men at an average gym chemically enhances his physique with anabolic steroids, the synthetic drug versions of testosterone.

Many people once believed that steroid use was limited to a few competitive athletes and bodybuilders—those who would risk their health to reach the top of their sport in order to claim titles, financial reward, and fame. This is not the case. Two of every three steroid users are recreational athletes with no intention of competing. The majority of steroid users take these drugs for personal reasons, seeking cosmetic improvement in their physiques. They just want to look good at the gym or buff on the beach. Most steroid users are 20 to 40 years of age, but 10 percent of users are teens. Surveys indicate that 2 to 5 percent of high school students are using these drugs. The steroid habit can start at a young age and continue for 10 years or more.

STEROID ACTION

Testosterone, the active ingredient in steroids, has two effects on the body: anabolic and androgenic. Testosterone's anabolic action builds body tissue by increasing lean muscle mass and bone density and reducing body fat. It ensures a positive nitrogen balance by stimulating protein synthesis and improving protein use. Testosterone's androgenic actions are responsible for the secondary sex characteristics that turn boys into men. All those changes that occur to boys during puberty—voice deepening, oily skin, growth of body and facial hair, development of male sex organs, and increased sex drive—occur because of a surge in teenage testosterone. A young adult male produces about 10 mg of testosterone each day, approximately 70 mg per week. The concentration of testosterone circulating in the blood of young males ranges from 300 to 1,000 nanograms per deciliter (ng/dl). The *average* level for adult men is about 500 ng/dl.

Author's note: This chapter is for educational purposes only. The use of anabolic drugs for nonmedical reasons without a doctor's prescription is illegal.

When discussing steroid doses, a distinction must be made between therapeutic doses aimed at restoring normal testosterone levels and the so-called supraphysiological doses used nonmedically for muscle building. The weekly dose for testosterone replacement is about 100 mg. According to scientific data, a weekly dose of at least 300 mg of testosterone is required for muscle building. This dose is equivalent to the combined testosterone levels of several men. Hence the term *supraphysiological*—more than the normal amount.

The results of scientific studies on testosterone are interesting. First, a 600 mg weekly dose of testosterone enanthate taken over a 10-week period produces a gain of 14 pounds (6.4 kg) in fat-free muscle mass and a 40 percent increase in strength. Second, testosterone-induced increases in muscle size are a result of muscle fiber hypertrophy, with an increase in the cross-sectional area of the muscle fibers. Third, these anabolic effects are dose dependant. Smaller doses of testosterone—125 mg per week or less—do not elevate the body's testosterone above normal levels. Only when the weekly dose of steroids is above 300 mg per week does the testosterone level climb above the normal range. A weekly 300 mg dose triples the average testosterone level, and a weekly 600 mg dose elevates the level up to six times the normal value. As a result, the 600 mg dose almost doubles the muscle fiber cross-sectional area, thereby increasing muscle size.

Testosterone exerts this anabolic effect by acting directly on the muscle itself. The hormone binds to androgen receptors in the muscle cell, switching on protein synthesis and inducing muscle growth. Testosterone also has several complementary anabolic actions elsewhere in the body. It stimulates the release of growth hormone and exerts an anticatabolic effect that slows protein breakdown. Testosterone also has a behavioral effect on the brain that might positively influence training intensity, thus increasing muscle strength.

As a result of recent research efforts, testosterone is now being prescribed as medical treatment for AIDS-related wasting disorders and as hormone replacement therapy in elderly men with low testosterone (the so-called male andropause). Testosterone has also been found to speed up the healing of muscle contusion injury and alleviate symptoms of depression in men.

STEROID DOSES AND REGIMENS

When it comes to discussing muscle-building steroid regimens, there's one big problem—the information is not based on scientific clinical investigation. Underground steroid regimens are anecdotal, based on word-of-mouth testimonies. In the absence of medical guidance, steroid users have been left to their own devices. Drug doses and regimens have been developed through trial and error, passed down by veteran users or through underground steroid manuals written by self-proclaimed steroid gurus.

So what's going on behind the closed doors of the locker room? A few years ago, I carried out a survey of the anabolic steroid regimens of 500 steroid users. The results revealed that the majority of users self-administered between 500 and 1,000 mg of steroids per week. Some bodybuilders who chose to be precise with their doses calculated them using this formula: 1 mg of steroid per kilogram of body weight per day. To achieve these megadoses, most users combined two or more types of steroids, a process known as stacking.

Steroids tend to be used in cycles lasting from 4 to 12 weeks. Regular steroid users allow a 4- to 6-week gap between cycles to clear the system. Approximately half the study group stated that their total annual steroid use amounted to more than six months each year. Some bodybuilders admitted to continuous steroid use for 52 weeks of the year without ever coming off the drugs.

In my survey, the most popular drug used was nandrolone decanoate, followed by injectable testosterones, such as Sustanon 250. Methandrostenolone (Dianabol) tablets came in third. Most steroid users choose a combination of injectable and oral steroids. Sample self-administered steroid regimens of new and veteran users, as reported during the survey, are shown in table 12.1. Even the most basic steroid cycle costs several hundred dollars.

Table 12.1 Sample Steroid Regimens (Self-Administered)

Cycle	Steroids	Dosage	Method of delivery	Time frame
Novice	Dianabol	25 mg/day	Oral	4-6 weeks
	Nandrolone decanoate	200 mg/week	Injection	
Mass	Sustanon	500 mg/week	Injection	4-6 weeks
	Nandrolone decanoate	400 mg/week	Injection	
Cutting	Testosterone propionate	300 mg/week	Injection	4-6 weeks
	Nandrolone decanoate	400 mg/week	Injection	
	Stanozolol	150 mg/week	Injection	
Off				4 weeks

THE POLYPHARMACY PROBLEM

Drug use by steroid users is not confined to anabolic steroids. Apparently, 9 out of 10 steroid users have a polypharmaceutical palate, taking a mix of muscle-shaping drugs in addition to stacking different brands of steroids. These steroid accessory drugs are used for a variety of reasons and can be grouped according to their desired effect.

Thermogenic fat-burning drugs, such as clenbuterol, ephedrine, and thyroid hormone, are common among steroid users. Nonsteroid anabolic agents, such as growth hormone and insulin, are gaining in popularity, particularly among competitive bodybuilders. Diuretics are used in an attempt to flush out subcutaneous body water before competition, and peculiar products such as Synthol are injected into lagging body parts to improve muscle symmetry and proportion. Medication is also taken to reduce side effects associated with steroid use. For example, the antiestrogen drug tamoxifen (Nolvadex) is used to prevent or treat steroid-induced gynecomastia (development of breast tissue). Human chorionic gonadotropin (HCG) is sometimes used to kick-start suppressed endogenous testosterone at the end of a steroid cycle to minimize muscle loss and withdrawal symptoms during the off cycle.

Many of these steroid accessory drugs are potentially more dangerous than the steroids themselves. The unsupervised use of insulin, diuretics, and thyroxine can precipitate a number of medical emergencies. It's a worrisome trend that healthy young bodybuilders take more drugs than their elderly grandparents with multiple medical ailments.

Recent data suggest that one in four steroid users is also taking growth hormone (somatotropin). So, what is it? Well, growth hormone (GH) is a substance made naturally in the pituitary gland, located at the base of the brain. It is an anabolic peptide hormone that stimulates growth of bone, cartilage, and muscle. It promotes protein synthesis, nitrogen balance, and fat loss. Synthetic drug versions of GH are effective only when delivered by injection. Sprays don't work because the GH molecule is too big to get into the bloodstream, and pills don't work partly because the drug is destroyed in the stomach. Because the natural production of GH decreases with age, GH drug therapy is gaining medical popularity as a form of hormone replacement in aging men. Although clinical studies have demonstrated some beneficial effects of GH replacement in elderly men, reporting gains in lean muscle mass, similar research has not yet been done on younger men with *normal* GH levels. From a scientific standpoint, we have little data on the effects of GH in young male athletes, so GH-using bodybuilders are essentially performing experiments on themselves. Reports indicate that bodybuilders using GH self-administer between 2 and 20 IUs per *day*. And those daily injections cost a lot of money! GH is not only costly, it's risky too. Its long list of possible complications include joint pains, injection-site reaction, fluid retention, headaches, muscle weakness, diabetes, hypothyroidism, carpal tunnel syndrome, abdominal distension, and leukemia. As with steroids, the use of GH without a doctor's prescription is illegal.

STEROID SIDE EFFECTS AND HEALTH RISKS

Because of their potential health risks, anabolic steroids are classed as illegal drugs and banned by many sporting organizations. Testosterone, the active ingredient in anabolic steroids, *does* work. It boosts muscle mass and turbocharges your sex drive. The problem is that testosterone, like any other drug, has potentially harmful effects.

How dangerous are these drugs? Are we to believe the shocking media reports of steroid-related deaths and the scare tactics employed by health professionals? If steroids are so dangerous, how come thousands of bodybuilders use them? Let's examine the hazards of steroid use in more detail.

There are many potential side effects associated with anabolic and androgenic steroids. Testosterone's anabolic action builds muscle, but its androgenic properties can adversely affect several body systems, including the cardiovascular, hormonal, reproductive, gastrointestinal, and nervous systems, as well as the skin. I've scanned the medical literature and compiled a list of all the possible complications of anabolic steroids. Take a look at table 12.2 for a summary of what can go wrong.

So, if you take anabolic steroids, what are the odds of developing a complication? The answer isn't straightforward because many factors determine the frequency and severity of side effects. In several short-term medical studies, a 600 mg weekly dose of testosterone caused no serious side effects in healthy adult men. Although this is a revelation in terms of steroid safety, we must interpret the data with caution. First, the studies lasted less than three months. Second, a 600 mg dose is moderate in comparison to what many bodybuilders use, often over long periods. One thing we do know is that the bigger the dose and the longer the duration of steroid use, the greater the health risk.

In surveys, more than 80 percent of steroid users report some kind of steroid-related complication. In other words, at least four of every five steroid users experience unwanted symptoms. These data imply that if you take large doses of anabolic steroids on a regular basis, your chance of experiencing a side effect is 80 percent or greater. The bottom line is that nearly all steroid users experience at

Table 12.2 Negative Effects of Anabolic Steroids

Heart	Liver	Skin
Elevated blood pressure	Liver toxicity	Acne
Raised cholesterol	Jaundice	Gynecomastia
Enlarged heart	Tumors	Stretch marks
Palpitations		Hair loss

Hormonal	Behavioral	Injection related
Libido changes	Mood swings	Bruising
Infertility	Aggression ("'roid rage")	Infection
In males:	Depression	Scar tissue
Small testes	Withdrawal	Nerve injury
Reduced sperm count	Addiction	HIV or hepatitis (sharing needles)
Impotence		
Enlarged prostate		
In females:		
Masculinization		
Voice deepening		
Menstrual irregularities		
Clitoris enlargement		
Reduced breast size		
In teens:		
Stunted growth		

least one of these common complications: acne, gynecomastia, testicle shrinkage, stretch marks, fluctuating sex drive, withdrawal symptoms, or drug dependence.

You might be thinking that these common steroid-induced complications are not real side effects—they're nothing more than a minor inconvenience. In fact, regular steroid users accept these problems as necessary evils in the pursuit of size, and rather than quit using steroids, they use other drugs to combat the unwanted symptoms. Some of the problems are reversible and disappear when steroid use is discontinued. Other effects, such as hair loss, stretch marks, and acne scars, can be permanent.

Testicle shrinkage   When you use anabolic steroids, your body senses a testosterone overload, and your testes stop making testosterone. Like many other body tissues, the testes function on the "use it or lose it" principle. When they're out of work, they shrink in size (atrophy). So while you're stomping around the mall trying on oversized shirts and baggy pants, you might also have to purchase a multipack of extra-small underwear. The only way to halt this period of self-induced testicular unemployment is to stop using steroids. Your testes will eventually regain their original size, but it will take six months or more of being steroid free. Some steroid users try to expedite this process by using such drugs as human chorionic gonadotrophin (Pregnyl) or clomiphene citrate (Clomid). These fertility drugs can kick-start sleeping testes back into action, but the effect is only temporary. The bottom line is that if you toy with testosterone, your testicles get tiny. You can't use juice and have a handful of big nuts at the same time.

Gynecomastia   The development of excessive breast tissue affects one in three male steroid users. What happens is that some of that extra testosterone circulating through your body gets converted to the hormone estrogen, which can lead to the development of a couple of female appendages. For many steroid users, this side effect is reversible—when they quit using the drugs, the gynecomastia disappears—but this isn't always the case. Treatment for gynecomastia is the antiestrogen drug tamoxifen (Nolvadex), 20 mg daily. This prescription-only medication can be used to treat gynecomastia or prevent it from occurring in the first place. Persistent cases of gynecomastia that resist drug treatment usually require surgical excision.

Skin changes   Testosterone is converted into dihydrotestosterone (DHT), a by-product that makes the skin more oily, which causes acne. DHT can also accelerate male-pattern baldness. The prescription drug finasteride (Propecia or Proscar) might help block the conversion of testosterone to DHT. Steroids can also affect skin elasticity, inflicting stretch marks as the muscles balloon in size.

Withdrawal   Steroid-induced problems don't end when you finish a steroid cycle. At least 70 percent of steroid users report symptoms of withdrawal after quitting the drug. Withdrawal symptoms include loss of muscle size and strength, fatigue, reduced sex drive, and depression. Because steroids suppress your own hormone production, when you discontinue the drugs, your testosterone level drops into your boots. That is, coming off the juice leaves you with the testosterone level of a toddler. It's no surprise that you feel as weak as a kitten when you stop taking steroids. Your muscles shrink, your strength falls off, and you lose interest in sex.

Addiction   The knee-jerk reaction to withdrawal is to score some more steroids pretty damn quick. You crave the rush of all that testosterone pumping through your veins, and this does represent a form of psychological (and physical) drug dependence. Sure, it's tough pedaling a bicycle to the gym when you're used to driving a tank—but you've got to step down sometime or risk devastating consequences.

Tendon injury   People once thought that anabolic steroids damaged tendons. Recent scientific evidence has shown this is not true. Anabolic steroids do not damage or weaken tendons. These drugs can make tendons mechanically stiffer and less elastic, but similar changes are induced in tendons by regular exercise. Anabolic steroids neither reduce tendon strength nor inflict any significant biochemical or anatomical alterations in tendon tissue. A word of caution, though. Anabolic steroids can increase muscular strength dramatically within a few weeks. Tendons, meanwhile, require longer to adapt (because they have a poorer blood supply). To avoid tendon injury, increase weight gradually to allow tendons time to get stronger.

Long-term risks   With chronic long-term steroid use, doses tend to increase and cycles become longer and more frequent. Eventually, some users take the drugs almost continuously for many years. The most severe consequences of long-term steroid use may be to your most vital organ—the heart. Steroids can cause the heart to enlarge abnormally, which impairs heart rhythm (palpitations) and function, leading to an increased risk of stroke, heart attack, and sudden death. This is no joke! The risk of death in long-term users of steroids is reported to be four times higher than in the normal population of nonusers. In other words, if you take steroids for several years, you may suffer an early death.

STEROID STICKS: INJECTION ISSUES

That guy at the gym who's the size of a gorilla might be big and strong, but don't congratulate him with a pat on the butt after his 600-pound (270 kg) bench press because his ass hurts from all those steroid needles. Needle injections are a big part of the steroid game. Nine of 10 steroid users inject muscle-building drugs; along with all those needle sticks comes a selection of injection-related problems.

Like most drugs, anabolic steroids can be taken by mouth or delivered via intramuscular injection. Tablets are a convenient way of taking medications—you simply pop them in your mouth and swallow. By contrast, injectable drugs require a needle, a syringe, and a sharp stick.

The side effects of steroids are similar for both tablet and injectable versions of the drug. Generally speaking, the health risks are predominantly dose related—the bigger the dose, the greater the risk. However, tablets and injections differ slightly when it comes to complications.

Tablets are potentially more harmful to the liver. Any oral drug absorbed from the gut passes through the liver before it's distributed elsewhere in the body. When taken in large doses by mouth, tablet versions of anabolic steroids can upset liver function. For this reason, many steroid users choose injectable forms of the drug to minimize toxic effects on the liver. Injectable versions of the drug are placed into muscle and released directly into the bloodstream, bypassing the liver. This means that larger doses can be injected without the liver taking a big hit. But there's a trade-off. Although the liver is partly spared drug toxicity, sticking a needle into your body is not without risk, especially if the person giving the injection has not been trained to perform the procedure. Injection problems are not necessarily related to the type of drug inside the syringe. They are purely the result of the needle stick. Common side effects of poor injection technique are pain, bruising, scar tissue buildup, nerve injury, infection or abscess, and HIV or hepatitis from sharing needles.

Intramuscular injection inflicts two forms of pain. The first is that sharp stick as the needle penetrates the skin. The second is a deep discomfort as the injection pushes the muscle fibers apart, creating a little pocket of fluid. The larger the volume of fluid, the greater the pain. Bigger muscles such as the buttocks and thighs can comfortably accommodate 2 to 3 ml of fluid. In smaller muscles, such as the shoulders, 1 ml is about the maximal limit of comfort. The fluid disappears as the drug is absorbed, but the site remains slightly damaged and inflamed from the needle stick for a while longer. If you inject into the same site within the space of a few days, you can cause a double-jeopardy situation. Double the fluid, double the damage, double the pain.

Needle size also influences the amount of pain. Larger-diameter needles cause more tissue damage than do narrower needles. Longer needles are more likely to damage an underlying nerve or blood vessel.

Every time a needle pierces muscle, a small amount of bleeding occurs. Under normal circumstances, this is not a problem, but if the needle hits a blood vessel, blood loss into the surrounding tissue can cause an unsightly (and painful) bruise, or hematoma. Much worse, injecting the drug directly into the bloodstream can cause a life-threatening embolism, stroke, or cardiac arrest. An injection-site bruise does not usually require treatment, but it can take a week or so to heal.

An injection needle actually *damages* muscle. As the stick plunges inside, it inflicts a tiny hole that heals by forming a scar. A small slither of scar tissue from one injection is no big deal, but repeated needle sticks eventually create a large area of scarring. Subsequent injections into this hard, gritty stuff become difficult and painful. Many bodybuilders don't realize that scar tissue is not normal muscle tissue; it doesn't contract or flex. It just sits there in the muscle like a golf ball.

Strange as it may seem, some bodybuilders attempt to fix holes in their physiques with a zap of oil. Injecting muscles with products such as Synthol gives an illusion of size but does not induce muscle growth. The fake size isn't muscle tissue—it's a bubble of oil, an injectable implant that doesn't contract. The muscle tissue becomes inflamed, eventually forming a bump of scar tissue that resembles a tumor of mutant muscle.

It's scary how bodybuilders play their own version of Russian roulette with steroid injections, blindly stabbing different body parts without knowing the location of nerves and blood vessels. Site injection is a common practice by bodybuilders. Steroids are injected directly into lagging muscle groups to induce a localized increase in size. The problem is most muscles are intimately adjacent to nerves, blood vessels, and other important anatomical structures. For instance, the radial nerve lies immediately under the triceps horseshoe, the sciatic nerve passes under the lower portion of your gluteals, and the axillary nerve lies beneath the deltoid muscle. If your misplaced needle hits an artery or vein, the extra blood loss creates a good-sized bruise. Striking a nerve with your needle feels like an electric shock. The damaged nerve can result in loss of feeling and muscle weakness.

Another possible side effect of poor injection technique is infection, which usually results from accidental contamination of a sterile needle, reusing needles, or sharing injection equipment or multidose vials with another person. All injections should be given using a sterile technique in a clean environment without contaminating the end of the needle. The locker room of your local gym does not qualify as a sterile area! Cleansing the skin with an alcohol swab can reduce the risk of infection. If the needle does get dirty after being removed from the sterile packaging, you run the risk of introducing a bacterial infection under your skin. This infection can develop into an abscess filled with pus, which usually needs to be lanced or surgically removed. Fake or counterfeit steroids that have not undergone proper sterilization can also increase the risk of bacterial infection. A more serious infection complication can arise from sharing needles. This hazardous practice risks the transmission of the HIV virus and hepatitis B or C.

STEROIDS LAB TESTS

Whether you are taking steroids legally or illegally, it's wise to get a regular health check from your physician. During the evaluation, it's important to mention any adverse reactions to steroids such as acne. The physical exam should include a blood pressure measurement and a check for other problems such as gynecomastia. Routine lab tests such as a complete blood count (CBC), cholesterol levels, and kidney and liver function tests are useful to screen for steroid-induced health problems. In some cases, abnormal findings may require further investigations and treatment. Table 12.3 highlights some of the more common laboratory abnormalities associated with steroid use. If any of your lab tests come back abnormal, your health is obviously being compromised by drug use, and perhaps your body is telling you it's time to quit.

Table 12.3 Laboratory Abnormalities in Steroid Users

Complete blood count (CBC)	Increased hemoglobin and red blood cells
Cholesterol levels	Decreased HDL ("good" cholesterol) Raised LDL ("bad" cholesterol)
Liver function tests	Raised liver enzymes
Hormone levels	Increased testosterone (on steroids) Decreased testosterone (off steroids)
Electrocardiogram (EKG)	Enlarged heart, rhythm disturbance
Echocardiogram	Impaired heart function
Prostate-specific antigen	Raised, with enlarged prostate
Semen analysis	Decreased sperm count

A WORD OF CAUTION

Although short-term use of low doses of testosterone may appear relatively safe, the potential health risks of long-term steroid use are still being researched. As the dose and duration of steroid use escalate, so do the health risks. Relatively minor side effects evolve into bigger problems, manifesting as irreparable heart or liver damage, high blood pressure, stroke, or heart attack. If everybody jumped off a cliff, would you follow them? Self-administering anabolic steroids is illegal and dangerous.

What follows is a list of the top 10 reasons *not* to take steroids. Although some of these risks may not apply to everyone, any would-be steroid user should think long and hard about the following consequences.

1. Anyone using anabolic steroids for nonmedical reasons is breaking the law.
2. Athletes taking steroids risk losing their opportunities to compete in sports.
3. Four out of every five steroid users experience side effects such as acne, gynecomastia, decreased libido, and hair loss.
4. Steroid use by teens can stunt growth.
5. Steroid use by females carries a high risk of permanent complications such as facial hair growth and voice deepening, even with short-term use.
6. Anabolic steroids upset normal hormone balance, causing withdrawal symptoms when the drugs are stopped, which can lead to addiction.
7. Long-term steroid use can cause heart abnormalities and an increased risk of death.
8. The bigger the dose of steroids, the bigger the health risks.
9. Drug use causes interpersonal problems in many aspects of social life, creating difficulties with relationships, family, and employment.
10. Illegally acquired steroids from bootleg sources are of questionable quality, content, and sterility.

The chances are good that at least one in five readers of this book have used, or considered using, anabolic steroids. If you choose to use these drugs, stick with lower doses and take adequate off cycles. Remember that bodybuilding is supposed to be a healthy pastime, not a fast track to an early demise. In the next chapter, we look at some of the nutritional supplements that offer a safe method of enhancing your physique.

Supplement Stack

In the same way that your exercise regimen evolves by climbing the ladder of intensity, your fuel intake can evolve with supplementation. However, keep the need for nutritional supplements in perspective. As the name suggests, these products are intended to supplement a balanced diet. They don't replace the need for food, nor do they compensate for a poor diet. Nevertheless, consuming the right food and the best supplements will improve efforts at muscle gain and fat loss. Enhancing your physique with nutritional supplements is a safer choice than chemical assistance with anabolic steroids.

The idea that certain substances enhance sporting performance is not new. In fact, the notion dates back to the first Olympic Games in 776 BC. Historical records describe some athletes using herbs and plant extracts to gain a competitive edge. Not so long ago, a protein shake meant a glass of whole milk with a few raw eggs thrown in. Over the past few decades, we have witnessed major developments in sport nutrition. Health food stores have become as commonplace as coffee shops, and the catalog of different products can be confusing. New must-have products are emerging so fast, it's tough to keep up.

Over the years, I have witnessed many products come and go. New supplements get hyped as the next best thing, only to disappear without a trace by your next birthday. Sadly, the quality of some supplements is questionable. We've all seen those amazing advertising claims that seem too good to be true. It's tough for consumers to distinguish fact from fiction, and we should not have to spend hours scanning the medical literature to determine whether a company's research claims are bogus. It isn't right that consumers are misled into parting with hard-earned cash for an overpriced product that is no more effective than powdered milk, particularly if that supplement could cause more harm than good.

If I were to list the thousands of products available on the market today, you'd have to sift through a compendium the size of a phone book. Instead, in this chapter I narrow my discussion to the supplements I believe are most useful for muscle building and fat loss.

There are six common reasons for using nutritional supplements:

1. To conveniently boost calories. Supplements are ready to eat anytime, anywhere.
2. To add fuel and increase protein intake.

3. To gain an ergogenic edge, boosting your workout performance.

4. To help burn fat and lose weight.

5. To provide a hormonal boost and help anabolism.

6. To provide additional benefits, such as preventing joint pain or vitamin deficiency.

As I mentioned, nutritional aids are intended to supplement your diet, not replace it. None of the products listed in this chapter is absolutely essential, but all of them can help build muscle and support fat loss. Based on efficacy and safety, the products currently available for bodybuilding purposes are summarized in table 13.1.

Table 13.1 Doctor's Bag of Supplements

Supplement	Comments
Meal-replacement products	Convenient source of nutrients. Useful when you don't have time to prepare (or eat) a meal.
Whey protein	Excellent source of high-quality protein to boost daily intake. Liquid formulations are easily digested and absorbed, making them ideal for refueling immediately after a workout.
Creatine	Enhances exercise performance and recovery. Increases muscle size and strength.
Fat burners	An aid to losing body weight.
Prohormones	Steroid precursors that convert to testosterone.
Glucosamine	Natural alternative to anti-inflammatory medication in the treatment and prevention of joint pain.
Multivitamins and minerals	Although vitamins and minerals will not directly help you build muscle or lose fat, supplementation ensures that you avoid dietary deficiencies.

I have put together a short list of the most effective supplements on the market today. Each product has qualified for inclusion based on its track record and scientific research. But keep three points in mind. First, the list contains only products that can help you build muscle and lose fat *legally*. I have not included products that are illegal or those not backed by scientific research. Nor have I included products that have other potential benefits such as improved sexual performance, restful sleep, or a reduced risk of colds and flu. This book is all about sculpting a better body, so the supplements are streamlined to this topic. Second, science is constantly moving forward. In the near future, new products might be added to this list, and some might be withdrawn. Third, laws differ from country to country, and although a substance may be banned in the United States, it can be legal in other parts of the world. The ones listed here are the most popular legal supplements available in the United States at the time of writing this chapter.

For convenience, for each product I answer the same four questions: What is it? Does it work? How much should I take? Is it safe?

MEAL-REPLACEMENT PRODUCTS

A meal-replacement product (MRP) does exactly what its name suggests. It provides a convenient way for you to consume all the nutrients you'd expect from a complete, healthy meal. The main advantage of a good MRP is convenience. It can be consumed anytime, anywhere, with minimal preparation. What's more, when you're outside of the home, you don't have to rely on traditional fast-food eateries, where the calorie content of the meal is an unknown quantity. The product label of a good-quality meal replacement tells you exactly what you're eating. MRPs are also generally cheaper than your average fast-food meal.

A good MRP should provide nutrients in the proportions you need, such as 50 percent protein, 40 percent carbohydrate, and 10 percent fat. It should also contain all the essential vitamins and minerals. The difference between a good bodybuilding MRP and other formulations is the relative content of protein and fat. Try to choose a product containing at least 30 grams of protein, with no more than a few grams of fat. Match the calorie content of the meal replacement with what you would expect from a regular meal—around 300 calories. MRPs are available in powder form (mixed with water), in ready-to-drink bottles, or in bars that look like candy bars.

MRPs are a reliable source of fast, convenient food. They are not directly ergogenic; they won't boost your workout performance. They will, however, enhance recovery by providing all the essential muscle-building nutrients. The liquid formulation is easily digested and more readily absorbed than a meal of solid food, so you won't feel bloated although your hunger will be satisfied.

Depending on your daily schedule, you can substitute an MRP for any meal. You should consume at least three meals of solid food each day, but an MRP is ideal for either of the other two meals, typically eaten at midmorning or midafternoon. As long as your MRP is from a reputable manufacturer, there's no cause for health concerns, but do make sure it's not loaded with fat calories.

PROTEIN

As discussed in chapter 2, protein is a component of all living cells and is essential for the growth and repair of body tissues. Although the foods mentioned in chapter 2, such as tuna and egg whites, are excellent sources of protein, preparing them can be inconvenient, and making them tasty sometimes means adding unwanted calories.

Alternatively, protein supplementation is a convenient way of increasing your intake and ensuring you get your daily requirement of amino acids. The most effective muscle-building supplements contain whey protein, which has a biological value (BV) of more than 100. To make protein supplements even more convenient, some products are packaged ready to drink or are available in the form of tasty bars.

To meet your daily protein requirement, each of your meals should contain at least 30 grams of protein. Your intestine will absorb 30 to 40 grams of protein per meal. If you want to stay lean, make sure your protein supplement is not loaded with extra carbohydrate or calories. Consuming 30 to 40 grams of protein with each meal is not harmful if you have good kidney function and you stay well hydrated.

CREATINE

Creatine is high-grade muscle fuel. After exercise, the muscle's supply of creatine is depleted, and it can take days to replenish the fuel store. Dietary supplementation with creatine boosts energy stores in muscle, enhancing recovery and exercise performance.

Creatine is probably the best legal supplement for gaining muscle mass and strength. In a recent review of scientific studies involving sport supplements, creatine came out on top of the list. Creatine has more research data documenting its ergogenic effects than other products on the market at this time. If you want the best bang for your buck, creatine may be your supplement of choice.

Expect to gain up to 10 pounds (4.5 kg) of muscle and increase your strength by 10 percent within several weeks of supplementing your diet with creatine. Creatine creates these results by enhancing energy stores in muscle, boosting muscle cell volume, increasing protein synthesis, and stimulating the release of growth hormone. As a result, exercise capability is improved and recovery time is quicker. Creatine supplementation has also been found to increase intramuscular insulin-like growth factor 1 (IGF-1). Gains in muscle size and strength are better when creatine is combined with whey protein, and the improvements are maintained for six weeks after supplementation is discontinued.

Consume a loading dose of 25 grams daily for the first three to five days, followed by a maintenance dose of 5 grams per day. With supplementation, the concentration of creatine is elevated by about 25 percent. This value reaches a peak after one week, indicating that the creatine level has reached a plateau. Once the fuel tank is full, consuming larger doses won't provide additional benefit. You can take your daily dose of creatine at any time during the day, but for the best effect, take it within an hour after your workout to take advantage of the anabolic window.

Most scientific studies have praised creatine's safety record, concluding that short-term use of this supplement is well tolerated in healthy young adults. However, creatine ingestion has been reported to cause cramps, dehydration, dizziness, stomach upset, and kidney problems. The main safety concern is that creatine possibly upsets the body's fluid balance, placing unwanted stress on the kidneys and liver. This remains a theoretical risk, however, because safety tests on creatine have failed to demonstrate any serious adverse effects. Overall, it appears that creatine does not cause harm to healthy young adults who use the recommended dosage. To ensure safety, it's wise to cycle your creatine use. For example, take it for 6 to 12 weeks, then go off it for 4 to 6 weeks to allow your body to return to normal. Creatine supplementation is not recommended in children, the elderly, or people with medical disorders.

FAT BURNERS

Supplements that promote fat loss are commonly called fat burners, thermogenic supplements, or lipotropic agents. These products can increase the body's natural fat-burning potential. They work via a process called thermogenesis, causing a natural elevation in your metabolic rate, allowing you to burn more calories while at rest. The more calories burned, the greater the weight loss.

Historically, fat burners combined the thermogenic properties of several ingredients, usually ephedrine, caffeine, and Aspirin (known as the ECA stack). For a more natural approach to fat loss, products then evolved to contain the *herbal* equivalents of ECA, namely ma-huang (ephedra), guarana (caffeine), and willow bark (Aspirin). Fat loss from ECA was likely the result of a combination of effects, including increased metabolic rate, raised body temperature, suppressed appetite, improved use of fats for energy, and greater exercise intensity. Ephedrine is a thermogenic agent that can convert excess calories into heat instead of fat. It also suppresses appetite. Caffeine promotes the use of fatty acids as an energy source during exercise so you can train harder longer. It also has a mild diuretic effect, which helps shed excess water, making the body appear leaner and tighter. Besides their fat-burning properties, both ephedrine and caffeine are stimulants that increase alertness, helping you exercise with greater intensity. Aspirin works in concert with ephedrine and caffeine to prolong the fat-burning effects in the body.

Because of safety and health concerns, ephedrine- and ephedra-containing products are now banned in many countries. Fat-loss supplements have therefore evolved again, and newer products are now ephedra free. Currently, the active ingredients in fat-loss supplements include natural extracts that are thought to support thermogenesis, enhance fat oxidation, and suppress appetite (table 13.2). The combinations of ingredients in weight-loss products vary, and the serving size differs in individual brands. Read the product label, and follow dosage instructions carefully. Start with the smallest serving size to monitor your own tolerance of the active ingredients. And remember, fat-loss agents work best when combined with a low-calorie, low-fat diet and regular aerobic exercise.

Table 13.2 Active Ingredients in Weight-Loss Supplements

Ingredient	Description
Caffeine	Supports thermogenesis; increases calorie expenditure and energy
Garcinia cambogia (hydroxycitric acid)	Believed to produce weight loss; appetite suppressant
Green and white tea	Supports thermogenesis; increases calorie expenditure
Hoodia	Appetite suppressant

The potential side effects of fat burners tend to arise from the stimulant effects of some ingredients (e.g., caffeine). Unwanted symptoms may include headache, sleeplessness, tremor, anxiety, dizziness, irregular heartbeat, behavioral changes, and high blood pressure. Weight-loss supplements are intended for use by healthy young adults. Clearly, these products are *not* suitable for people who suffer from medical conditions such as high blood pressure, irregular heartbeat, recurrent headaches, stroke, or diabetes. Fat burners made by reputable companies should have a statement clearly warning consumers on the product label. Some people react more strongly to caffeine than others, and there is an individual susceptibility to adverse effects. If you are concerned about the risks of using weight-loss supplements, consult your doctor beforehand. Should you suffer any unusual symptoms while using a fat burner, stop using the product, and seek medical advice.

In the United States, weight-loss supplements are constantly under the scrutiny of the Food and Drug Administration. What might be a popular formulation today might be deemed (relatively) unsafe tomorrow. Make your own informed decision before using a product, and if in doubt just stick with diet and exercise for fat loss.

Hey, I lost seven pounds (3 kg) in body weight this week. Do you want to know how I did it? Well, I did not diet, and I did not take any supplements. All I did was simply jog for 20 minutes (about two miles or 3 km) a day for seven days.

PROHORMONES

Steroid prohormones such as androstenedione, norandrostenedione, and dehydro epiandrosterone (DHEA) are precursors of, or building blocks for, testosterone. When consumed, prohormones convert to testosterone inside your body. In theory, these supplements are a natural method of increasing testosterone levels. Research indicates that a 300 mg dose of the prohormone androstenedione can increase testosterone levels. However, whether this effect benefits muscle size and strength is not yet proven. The recommended dose of androstenedione is 300 mg daily. Lower doses do not raise testosterone levels. Prohormones are not free of potential problems. First, there's the issue of safety. Research studies investigating the effects of androstenedione given to healthy adult men in daily doses of 300 mg for up to 12 weeks have found the product to be relatively safe. However, concerns exist that prohormones produce side effects similar to anabolic steroids, such as acne. The ingested prohormone can also convert into the female steroid estrogen, and some male users have developed gynecomastia (female breast tissue). For women, there's a risk of developing masculine features (hirsutism), and in children there's a possibility of stunted growth. A second problem relates to drug testing. If you're taking prohormones, your urine might test positive for anabolic steroids. And finally, prohormones are now illegal in the United States and have been withdrawn from the stores.

GLUCOSAMINE

Glucosamine is a naturally occurring amino sugar that plays an important role in the cartilage that cushions human joints. Glucosamine is a building block for the large molecules that attract and hold water inside cartilage, providing better shock absorption. Unfortunately, cartilage wears down over time, and the body's ability to replace it slows or ceases. This can result in arthritis and painful, stiff joints. Glucosamine acts as a joint saver, helping maintain the cartilage cushion and lubrication inside your joints, much like oiling the moving parts of a machine.

As your body gets older, the cartilage cushion inside your joints wears down. The process is similar to tire wear as the mileage on your vehicle increases. Over time, lifting heavy weights can injure joints and increase the rate of cartilage loss. As the years go by, glucosamine supplementation may help slow down the wear and tear inside your joints as well as help relieve symptoms of joint pain. The recommended dose of glucosamine is 1,500 mg daily. The benefit of other additives, such as chondroitin, are less proven at this time.

According to current scientific knowledge, glucosamine supplementation is safe. Few side effects have been reported with glucosamine use. Because it's a naturally occurring substance, it's less toxic than other drugs used to treat joint pain and arthritis.

Herbs

Herbal remedies seem to be popular nowadays. According to surveys, an estimated 12 percent of the U.S. population take herbal supplements such as echinacea, ginseng, Gingko biloba, and St. John's wort. Whether or not these herbs provide any significant health benefits remains the subject of scientific debate, and the true incidence of side effects is unknown. Because these herbs are classified as dietary supplements, they are exempt from the laws that regulate regular medications. As a consequence, the potency of herbal medications is widely variable, and this presents a tough hurdle when it comes to collecting hard scientific data on the subject. Here's what we do know about some common herbs.

Echinacea allegedly enhances the immune system and is used to prevent colds and flu. But long-term usage may be harmful, *suppressing* immunity and actually increasing the risk of certain infections.

Ginseng is thought to protect the body against stress, and Gingko biloba is used to improve mental function. However, both herbs can adversely affect blood clotting, increasing the risk of bleeding and resulting in easy bruising. Users of ginseng and Gingko would be wise to stop taking these herbs seven days before undergoing surgery to avoid excessive bleeding.

St. John's wort is used as a natural antidepressant to elevate mood. But this herb can block the action of certain drugs used to treat medical disorders as well as some agents used during surgery and anesthesia.

Despite a lack of high-quality clinical studies, it seems that some herbs may help promote health, but their long-term effects remain unknown. One final thought: Be sure to mention your herbal habits to your doctor, surgeon, or anesthesiologist—your life might depend on it.

MULTIVITAMINS AND MINERALS

Vitamins and minerals are essential dietary micronutrients. They serve many functions in the body, and dietary deficiency can result in ill health. These micronutrients don't directly help build muscle or reduce body fat, but an adequate supply of dietary vitamins and minerals is necessary for optimal athletic performance (see chapter 2).

A well-balanced diet provides all the vitamins and minerals you need. If you suspect your diet is not consistently well balanced, a simple solution to avoid deficiency is to take a daily multivitamin and mineral supplement. There are many inexpensive multivitamin and mineral formulations available at most health food and drug stores. Usually, one tablet per day provides the recommended daily intake of all the essential micronutrients—just be sure to check the label carefully.

GOODIES OR GIMMICKS?

Here are a few tips on how to distinguish good supplements from bad and effective nutritional aids from fads.

Tip 1 Select brands made by a reputable company with a track record in sport nutrition. Larger companies that have been in the business for many years are more likely to produce legitimate products than are smaller, relatively new companies. Reputable manufacturers should perform stringent safety checks on the ingredients contained in their products.

Tip 2 Be cautious of new products that emerge overnight and claim to be the next best thing. It can take years of clinical research to prove the benefit of new products.

Tip 3 Beware of advertising claims that appear too good to be true. Frequently, the references cited in these ads don't exist. If the name of the scientific journal is abbreviated beyond recognition or if the reference is not written in English, there's a good chance the source is fictitious. Many times a reference or journal article is not listed at all. Another suspicious feature is when the research was not performed on humans. It's just not possible to predict the effect a product will have on human subjects if it's been tested only on other species.

Tip 4 Be cautious with products available exclusively through mail order or the Internet. Why aren't these products for sale in retail health stores? Sometimes the reason is that the product is illegal. There have been reports that some so-called natural anabolic supplements are contaminated with illegal, potentially dangerous substances. If this is the case, you're not only risking your health by ordering these products but also breaking the law.

Tip 5 If in doubt, give the product a tryout. Do your own research study. Buy a small container of the product, and take it as directed on the label. Continue your current exercise routine and nutrition program; the only change you have made is adding the trial product. After a month or so, assess whether the product did what it was supposed to. Did you get stronger? Did you gain muscle? Did you lose body fat? Did you suffer side effects? If you did not get the results you were expecting from the product, it probably does not work for you.

Laws change, and scientific knowledge evolves. What's legal today may be illegal tomorrow. And what is believed to be safe at the present time may be found to be a health risk in the future. During the past decade, we have witnessed the banning of ephedra and prohormones for safety reasons.

On a final note, please remember that nutritional supplements are intended to *supplement* a healthy diet and regular exercise. Should you become obsessed with supplements, then you are missing the point. Throughout this book, I provide you with a strong scientific foundation to create effective exercise and nutrition programs to sculpt your body and achieve your physique goals. Nutritional supplements are merely an optional extra. Remember: Keep it simple and safe!

Hybrid Hard Body Program

In part II of this book, we fire up the power tools for maximizing muscle mass. In part III, we rip open the complete package for fat loss. So far in part IV, we've unveiled the trade secrets of advanced bodybuilding. Now we combine all this knowledge and transform your physique to its maximum potential.

If you're looking to forge the ultimate physique, this plan is for you. The hybrid hard body workout combines 30 of the most effective muscle-shaping exercises into a four-day split-training routine. I have included a couple of cardio sessions in the weekly schedule to tease off that fat layer to showcase your hard-earned muscle. The hard body diet provides enough nutrients to fuel muscle growth, while careful calorie control starves your fat stores.

PROGRAM OVERVIEW

The hybrid system is a blend of techniques, a combination of bodybuilding styles that simultaneously stimulates muscle growth and promotes fat loss. In effect, with the hybrid system you get the best elements of the mass generator program (chapter 7) and the body fat blitz program (chapter 10) and then some.

Workout Plan

The hybrid hard body program is an advanced high-intensity body sculpting system designed for simultaneous muscle gain and fat loss. This program is best suited for the advanced bodybuilder. For those of you with less gym experience, I recommend that you spend a few months developing the basic techniques outlined in the previous two programs. If your primary need is muscle mass, use the mass generator program (chapter 7) to build a solid foundation of muscle before moving on to the hybrid hard body program. If your primary need is fat loss, use the body fat blitz program (chapter 10) before you progress to developing your body further.

The hybrid hard body program emphasizes high-intensity training. Perform three sets of each exercise, using weights equivalent to 65 to 75 percent of your one-rep maximum. After an initial warm-up set of 12 reps, increase the weight on the second set so that your muscles fatigue after 10 reps. For the final work set, add more weight and squeeze out 8 reps to failure. To make your muscles work hard, keep your rest intervals short—take 30 seconds of rest between the first two sets, 45 seconds between the next two sets, and 60 seconds before the final heavy set.

To gain the maximum benefit from this program, incorporate the high-intensity techniques in chapter 11. Most of the machine-based exercises in this program make it easy to train beyond failure using drop sets, forced reps, and negative reps. Still take the necessary safety precautions, and use a spotter.

Here's how the hybrid hard body four-way split-training system works. Session 1 involves the chest, triceps, and abs. Session 2 works the back, biceps, and forearms. Session 3 targets the quads, hamstrings, and calves. Session 4 works the shoulders, trapezius, and abs. This sequence groups body parts that share similar exercise biomechanics. For example, in session 1 the *push* exercises for the chest also recruit and warm up the triceps. Similarly, in session 2, the *pull* exercises for the back muscles recruit and warm up the biceps and forearm muscles. In both sessions, the smaller muscle is already pumped and ready for action when its turn comes. The leg muscles have session 3 all to themselves; being the largest muscle group, the quadriceps are hit first in the sequence. The shoulder muscles are trained at the end of the week in session 4 so that the muscles are rested after their assistance work with the pressing exercises in session 1. To achieve complete muscular development, the muscles of the shoulder need their own designated session. You'll be strengthening the muscles of the rotator cuff, shaping all three heads of the deltoid, and building the trapezius muscles. The abs, obliques, and serratus muscles are worked in both sessions 1 and 4. I've chosen a sequence of exercises that hit these muscles from all angles, helping you develop a tight midsection and six-pack.

In this program, you exercise each major muscle group once every seven days. Remember that your muscles need five to seven days to fully recover from an intense weights workout. Space your four workout sessions evenly during the week—for example, Monday, Tuesday, Thursday, and Friday. Larger muscles such as the chest, shoulders, back, and quads are each assigned three exercises; and, as a general rule, an isolation exercise is used to prime the muscle before compound movements. Each exercise hits the muscle from a different angle. Targeting different sections of the larger muscles ensures more complete muscular development.

During each 45-minute workout, you push yourself *hard* to achieve your potential. By the third set of each exercise, you should be lifting the heaviest possible weight for eight repetitions to failure, using flawless form. For at least one exercise per body part, you'll train beyond failure, using one or more of the high-intensity techniques in chapter 11.

As you gain experience using this program, feel free to change, add, or subtract exercises to meet your own needs and preferences. The exercises described in all three programs in this book are interchangeable. Just make sure your exercise combinations hit the larger muscle groups from different angles to ensure proportioned development. Don't add too many extra exercises, or you'll risk overtraining (see chapter 17).

Calorie-burning cardiorespiratory exercise is also included in this program. If you want that hard body look, you need to keep your body fat low. As I've mentioned, you won't see those rippling muscles or that shredded six-pack unless your body fat is below 10 percent. You should do two 30-minute sessions of continuous, low-resistance cardio on two of the days you're not lifting. Work hard enough to maintain your heart rate in the target zone (70 percent of your maximum heart rate—calculate your target heart rate by subtracting your age from 220 and multiplying by .7).

The type of aerobic exercise you do is up to you. Choose from walking, jogging, cycling, stair climbing, jumping rope, or swimming. It's more challenging if you vary the aerobic exercise, selecting a different activity for each cardio session. For example, cycle on a stationary bike during one session, then walk or jog on the treadmill during the other session.

Nutrition Plan

To gain muscle and lose body fat at the same time, consume roughly the same amount of calories that you burn each day. In other words, keep your daily calorie intake close to your maintenance requirement (body weight in pounds × 10, or body weight in kilograms × 22). You want to provide enough calories for muscle growth but force your body to get its additional energy through burning fat stores. The process might need some fine-tuning as you go along. Monitor your progress in terms of muscle gain and fat loss on a weekly basis. If you wish to gain more muscle mass, add 5 percent to your estimated daily calorie requirement; if you need to lose more body fat, subtract 5 percent from your estimated value. Adapting the program to meet your needs as they evolve is essential if you want continued progress.

To prevent excess carbohydrate from being stored as fat, the nutrient ratio of your diet should favor protein. Divide your food sources as 50 percent protein, 40 percent carbohydrate, and 10 percent fat.

The 1,800-calorie sample meal plan in table 14.1 is a rough guide for someone who weighs 180 pounds (82 kg), based on the estimated daily maintenance value (body weight in pounds × 10). If this person needs more muscle mass, he would add 5 percent to this value for a daily intake of 1,800 + 90, or 1,890 calories. On the flip side, if he needs to shed more body fat, he would subtract 5 percent (90 calories) from the maintenance value, which means consuming 1,710 calories per day.

Adjusting the sample meal plan to your weight is easy, based on the fact that 1 gram of protein is four calories, 1 gram of carbohydrate is four calories, and 1 gram of fat is nine calories. Keeping the nutrient ratio at 50 percent protein and 40 percent carbohydrate, 100 calories equals 15 grams of protein (60 calories) plus 10 grams of carbohydrate (40 calories). To increase or decrease the calorie content to match your body weight, add or subtract these amounts from the sample meal plan.

Adjust your protein intake by changing the amount of protein powder you add to your midafternoon snack or changing the number of egg whites you eat at breakfast (one egg white contains 6 grams of protein). Similarly, by adjusting your portions of pasta, potato, or rice at lunch and dinner, you can easily increase or decrease your intake of carbohydrate.

Remember that the nutrition values in the sample meal plan (table 14.1) are only approximate. Check nutrition labels on the products you buy because values vary among brands.

As mentioned, the 1,800-calorie sample meal plan is a rough guide for someone who weighs 180 pounds. Adjust the content of the sample meal plan to your body weight, using table 14.2. And remember, as your body weight changes, so should your calorie intake.

Some of the dietary supplements listed in chapter 13 can also aid your progress in the hybrid hard body program. In particular, creatine helps build muscle mass; a fat burner can help tease off unwanted body fat.

Table 14.1 Hybrid Hard Body Sample Meal Plan

Breakfast	Egg white scramble: Mix five egg whites with 1 tbsp of nonfat milk. Cook in a nonstick pan coated with nonfat cooking spray. Serve on one piece of whole-wheat toast. Drink one cup of black coffee or water. Calories: 320
Midmorning snack	Meal-replacement drink: Mix one sachet of a meal-replacement powder with 12 oz (360 ml) of cold water in a blender. Calories: 340
Lunch	Tuna meal: Microwave one medium-size potato. Steam a portion of green beans. Serve with one can of water-packed tuna sprinkled with lemon juice. Drink water. Calories: 260
Midafternoon snack	Protein drink: Mix two servings/scoops of whey protein powder with 4 oz (120 ml) water and 4 oz nonfat milk. Add one whole banana. Blend at high speed for 30 seconds. Calories: 300
Dinner	Chicken meal: Prepare a skinless chicken breast by squeezing lemon juice over it. Grill until cooked. Serve with a portion of steamed brown rice and broccoli. 1 tbsp of tomato ketchup is optional. Calories: 380
Late-evening snack	Eat a low-carbohydrate protein bar. Calories: 290
Daily values (approximate)	Protein: 225 g (900 cal), 50% Carbohydrate: 180 g (720 cal), 40% Fat: 20 g (180 cal), 10% Total calories: 1,800

Table 14.2 Maintenance Daily Calorie Intake Based on Body Weight (Hybrid Hard Body)

Body weight (lb)	Body weight (kg)	Calories per day	Protein	Carbohydrate	Fat
220	100	2,200	275 g (1,100 cal)	220 g (880 cal)	24 g (220 cal)
200	91	2,000	250 g (1,000 cal)	200 g (800 cal)	22 g (200 cal)
180	82	1,800	225 g (900 cal)	180 g (720 cal)	20 g (180 cal)
160	73	1,600	200 g (800 cal)	160 g (640 cal)	18 g (160 cal)
140	64	1,400	175 g (700 cal)	140 g (560 cal)	16 g (140 cal)

Nutrient ratio: 50% protein, 40% carbohydrate, 10% fat
Calorie values: 1 g protein = 4 calories; 1 g carbohydrate = 4 calories; 1 g fat = 9 calories
Daily calorie intake = body weight in pounds × 10 *or* body weight in kg × 22

Progress Measurements

Monitoring your progress is essential because fine-tuning your workouts and diet is key to advanced bodybuilding. Measure your body weight using a scale, and take body measurements—chest, waist, arm, thigh, and calf circumference—with a tape measure. Measure body fat percentage using a skinfold caliper. Following the manufacturer's instructions, record the skin thickness at three sites on your body, usually the upper arm, waist, and thigh. Calculate the average reading by adding all three measurements and then dividing by 3. You can also check your progress in the mirror. Check if each muscle group is developing in proportion. Lagging muscle groups might need more attention (see chapter 15). If you want that athletic V-shape taper, be sure to work your side deltoids and those outer lats, and narrow that waist by losing body fat. As you gain or lose body weight, adjust your calorie intake accordingly.

Measure muscle strength by recording the maximum weight you can lift for six repetitions during the last set of each exercise. The stronger the muscle becomes, the bigger it grows. The larger your muscle mass, the more fat you'll burn. To continue gaining size and strength, increase the weight on each exercise by 5 percent every two weeks.

Measure fitness during an aerobic exercise of your choice, such as cycling or jogging. Monitor how long you can sustain your heart rate at 70 percent of its maximum value. A person of average fitness should be able to sustain 70 percent maximum heart rate for 20 minutes (maximum heart rate equals 220 minus age in years multiplied by .7). Each week, aim to increase your cardio time by 10 minutes or increase your target heart rate by 5 percent (but no higher than 85% of your maximum heart rate). The harder you work for 30 minutes, the more calories you'll burn. The more calories you use, the more fat you lose.

Results

After six weeks on this program, you should gain three to four pounds (1.4-1.8 kg) of muscle and lose three pounds of body fat. You'll add an inch (2.5 cm) to your chest, lose an inch from your waist, and boost your arm and thigh circumference by half an inch (1.25 cm). As a result of this simultaneous muscle gain and fat loss, you should experience a 10 percent increase in strength and a 3 percent drop in body fat. Because you'll be gaining muscle and losing fat simultaneously, your body weight might not change much within six weeks on this program. Don't be alarmed—your gain in muscular weight is being offset by the loss of body fat. Your body measurements and body fat percentage are better indicators of your progress than are changes in your body weight.

HYBRID HARD BODY EXERCISE PROGRAM

Routine: Four-way split
Cycle: Four days per week weight training, two days cardio
Schedule: Monday, Tuesday, Thursday, Friday, plus two sessions for cardio
Goal: Muscle gain and fat loss
Detail: 3 sets of 12, 10, 8 reps
Rest interval: 30 to 60 sec
Workout time: 45 min

Chest, Triceps, and Abs Monday	
Chest	Machine chest fly
	Machine incline press
	Decline bench press
Triceps	Triceps dip
	One-arm triceps push-down
Abs	Rope crunch
	Cable side crunch

Legs Thursday	
Quadriceps	Leg extension
	Leg press
	Machine squat
Hamstrings	Leg curl
	Straight-leg deadlift
Calves	Seated calf raise
	Straight-leg calf raise

Back, Biceps, and Forearms Tuesday	
Back	Reverse-grip pull-down
	Dumbbell row
	Lumbar extension
Biceps	Preacher curl
	Concentration curl
Forearms	Barbell wrist curl
	Reverse wrist curl

Cardio Wednesday	
Cardio	Exercise of choice (30 min)

Shoulders and Abs Friday	
Rotator cuff	External rotation
	Internal rotation
	Cable lateral raise
Deltoids	Machine upright row
	Rear deltoid fly
	Front deltoid raise
Trapezius	Shrug
Abs	Machine crunch
	Bench leg raise

Cardio Saturday	
Cardio	Exercise of choice (30 min)

CHEST

Machine Chest Fly

This is a variation of the dumbbell chest fly (chapter 7) using a machine with either a hand grip or elbow pads. The chest fly machine is better suited to techniques of high intensity. Sit on the fly machine with the seat positioned so that the handles are at shoulder level (figure 14.1a). Grab the handles and squeeze them together until they're touching in front of you (figure 14.1b). Pause momentarily to contract your pecs forcibly before resisting back to the full stretch. Do not allow your hands to pass behind the plane of your body. Keep your elbows nearly straight and just below shoulder level at all times.

▶ **CHECK IT!** If your upper pecs are small relative to the rest of your chest, substitute this exercise with incline dumbbell flys. If your lower pecs need more attention, perform cable crossovers instead.

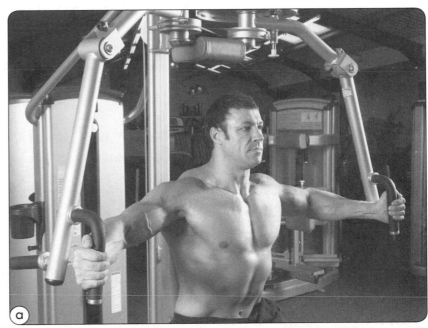

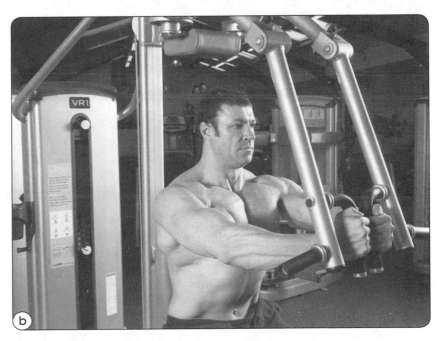

Figure 14.1 Machine chest fly: *(a)* Sit at the machine; *(b)* squeeze handles in front of chest.

Machine Incline Press

Place an adjustable exercise bench beneath the bar of a Smith machine; tilt the backrest to an angle of 30 to 45 degrees (head up). Before you load the machine with weight, lie back on the bench and check the trajectory of the bar. Position the bench so that the bar touches the midpoint of your chest when lowered. Position your feet firmly on the floor. Take an overhand grip on the barbell, palms turned forward, hands slightly wider than shoulder-width apart. Release the bar from the uprights; hold the bar above your chest with arms extended (figure 14.2a). Begin the repetition by bending your elbows.

Lower the weight slowly to the midpoint of your chest, just above the nipple line (figure 14.2b). Inhale as you lower the weight. Let the bar touch your chest, and hold for one second. Then push the weight vertically upward to the start position. Hold the bar while contracting your pecs, then repeat. You can perform this exercise using a barbell (chapter 7), using a pair of dumbbells (chapter 10), or on any incline press machine.

▶ **CHECK IT!** Hold the bar just short of lockout on the way up to keep tension on the chest muscles.

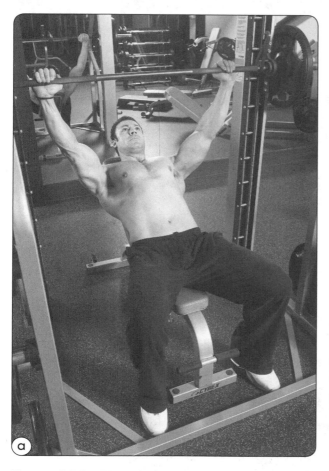 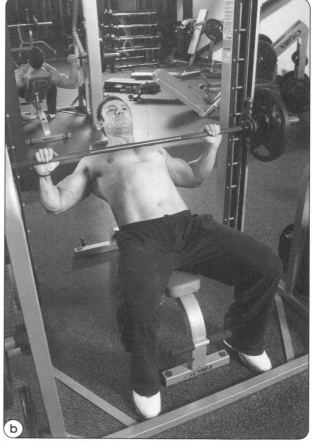

Figure 14.2 Machine incline press: *(a)* Hold the bar above your chest; *(b)* lower the bar.

CHEST

Decline Bench Press

Position an adjustable decline bench at an angle of 25 to 30 degrees in relation to the ground. Lie supine on the bench with a dumbbell in each hand. Hook your feet under the ankle pads. Press the dumbbells up until your elbows are fully extended over your chest, palms turned forward (figure 14.3*a*). From the start position, lower the dumbbells vertically downward by bending your elbows down and back. Keep the dumbbells in line with your palms turned forward. The weights should travel perpendicular to the floor. Lower the dumbbells until they are beside your chest at nipple level (figure 14.3*b*). Press the weights vertically upward back to the start position. Squeeze the pec muscles as the dumbbells touch in the lockout position. Hold one second and repeat. You can also do this exercise using the bar on the Smith machine.

▶ **CHECK IT!** Don't set the bench at a steep angle, or you'll work your triceps more than your chest.

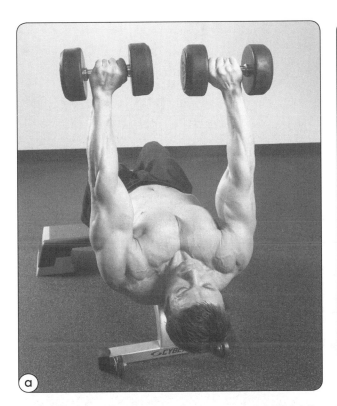 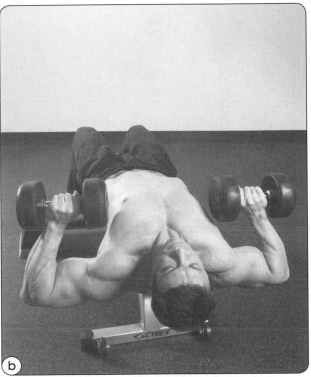

Figure 14.3 Decline bench press: *(a)* Hold the dumbbells over your chest; *(b)* lower the dumbbells to your chest.

Triceps Dip

Perform this exercise seated in the triceps push-down machine. Grab the handles with your palms turned in. In the start position, your elbows should bend to 90 degrees, with your upper arms parallel to the floor (figure 14.4a). Push the weight down until your arms are fully straight and your elbows lock out (figure 14.4b). Contract your triceps momentarily, then slowly return the weight to the start position and repeat. Alternatively, you may perform triceps dips on the parallel bar apparatus.

▶ **CHECK IT!** Keep your torso upright to focus effort on the triceps; if you lean forward, your chest muscles contribute to the movement.

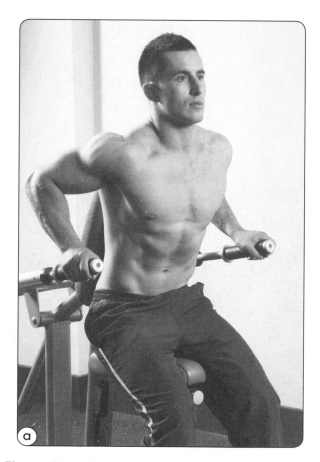 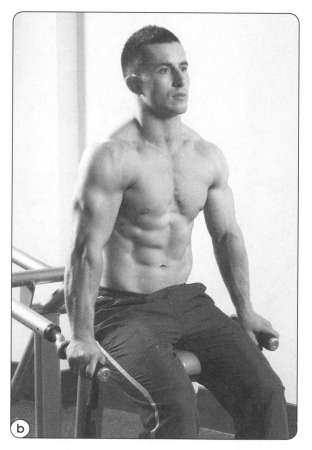

Figure 14.4 Triceps dip: *(a)* Sit in the machine and grasp the handles; *(b)* push the weight down.

One-Arm Triceps Push-Down

Attach a handle to the cable of a high pulley machine. Grab the handle in one hand with an underhand grip, palm facing upward. Position your upper arm perpendicular in relation to the floor, with your elbow fully bent (figure 14.5a). From the start position, straighten your arm, pushing the handle down. Keep your upper arm fixed during this exercise, restricting motion exclusively to your elbow. Hold the lockout position momentarily, contracting your triceps muscle (figure 14.5b). Then slowly return the handle to the start position and repeat. After you've completed the set number of reps with one arm, do the same with your opposite arm.

▶ **CHECK IT!** Keep your upper arms stiff so that motion occurs only at the elbows.

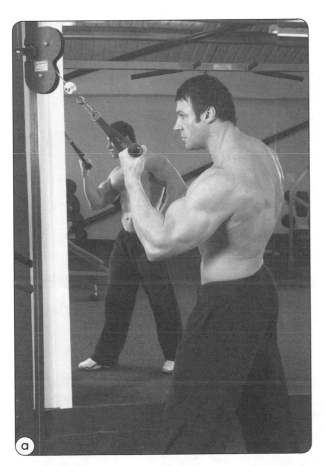 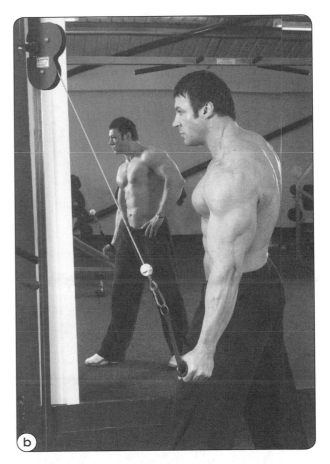

Figure 14.5 One-arm triceps push-down: *(a)* Hold the handle with your elbow bent; *(b)* push down toward the floor.

Rope Crunch

Connect a rope attachment to the cable of a high pulley and kneel on the floor beneath it, holding the ends of the rope in your hands. Pull the rope down and hold it behind your head (figure 14.6a). From this position, contract your abs to curl your torso down (figure 14.6b). Restrict movement exclusively to bending your spine. Your elbows should come down and back toward your knees, but the position of your hands and shoulders should not change. Hold momentarily to contract your abs on completion of the crunch, then slowly return to the start position and repeat. If you don't have access to a cable pulley machine, do decline sit-ups (chapter 7) as a substitute.

▶ **CHECK IT!**   Keep tension on the abs as you return to the start position, and avoid arching your lower back.

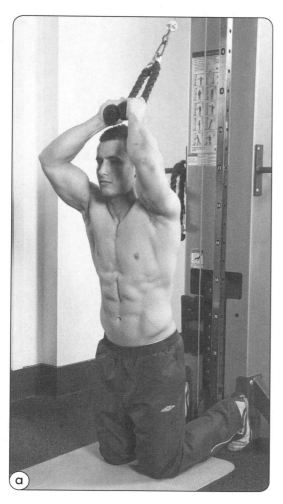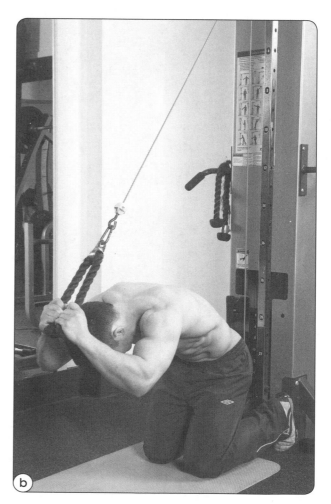

Figure 14.6   Rope crunch: *(a)* Hold the rope behind your head; *(b)* curl your torso.

Cable Side Crunch

Attach a handle to the high pulley of a cable machine. Grab the handle with one hand, and kneel on the floor beneath the pulley. Hold the handle close to the side of your head with your elbow bent (figure 14.7a). Crunch downward, directing your elbow to the opposite knee (figure 14.7b). Restrict movement exclusively to bending your spine. The angle of your arm at the shoulder should not change. Hold the side crunch position momentarily, squeezing your oblique muscles—feel them contract with your free hand. Then slowly return to the start position and repeat. After completing the set number of reps, switch hands and work the opposite side. You can also do this exercise in a standing position.

If you don't have access to a cable pulley, do twisting sit-ups (chapter 10) as a substitute to work the serratus and oblique muscles.

▶ **CHECK IT!**   During this exercise, feel the oblique muscles contracting with your free hand.

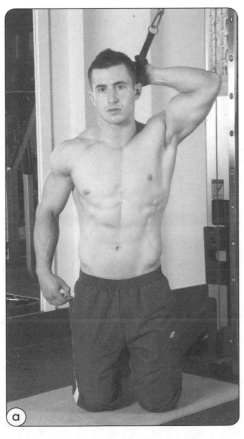 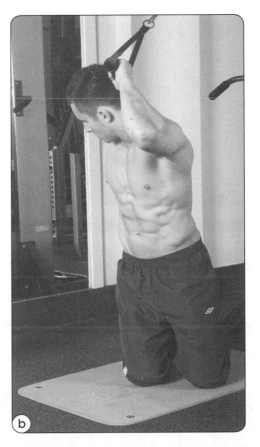

Figure 14.7   Cable side crunch: (*a*) Hold the handle adjacent to your head; (*b*) crunch down toward the opposite knee.

Reverse-Grip Pull-Down

Sit at a cable pull-down machine facing inward; position your thighs under the knee pads. Grasp the bar with a reverse underhand grip, palms turned toward you. Position your hands slightly less than shoulder-width apart. With your arms fully extended overhead, lean your torso back about 30 degrees from the vertical plane (figure 14.8a). Begin the repetition by pulling the bar down to the top of your chest (figure 14.8b). Think of your hands as hooks. Make your upper back muscles do the work, pulling your elbows down and back. Hold the bar above your collarbone for one second, contracting the latissimus muscles. Then slowly return the weight to the start position.

If you don't have access to a pull-down machine, you can do the same movement using a chin-up bar.

▶ **CHECK IT!** Don't pull the bar *below* collarbone level. Avoid leaning back too far, and don't pull the weight down with momentum.

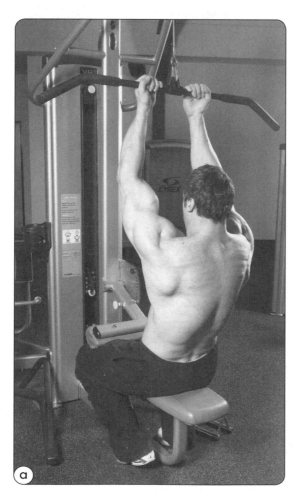 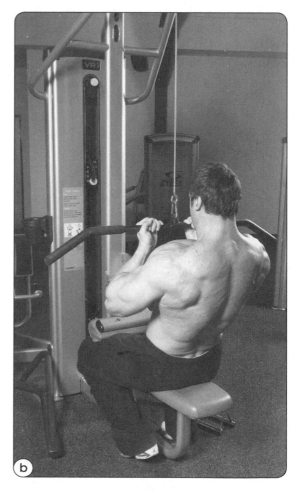

Figure 14.8 Reverse-grip pull-down: *(a)* Take an underhand grip on the bar; *(b)* pull the bar to your chest.

Dumbbell Row

Stand alongside a flat exercise bench. Rest one knee on the bench and lean forward, supporting your torso with the arm nearest the bench. Your back should be straight and just above parallel to the floor. Reach down and pick up a dumbbell with your free hand. Hold the weight with your arm extended vertically downward so that the dumbbell is parallel to the bench (figure 14.9a). From the start position, bend the elbow and pull the weight vertically upward until the dumbbell is level with your torso (figure 14.9b). Pause for a second at the top, contracting your upper back muscles, and then slowly lower the weight down to the start position without touching the ground. Repeat. Keep your forearm hanging straight down throughout the movement. After you complete the planned number of reps, switch positions and continue the set using the opposite arm.

You can do the row exercise using a barbell (chapter 7) or in a seated position using a low-pulley cable (chapter 10). My personal favorite is the seated row machine, with a built-in chest pad that reduces the strain on the lower back. Performing the row exercise using one arm at a time affords a more satisfying squeeze in the latissimus muscle.

> ▶ **CHECK IT!** Look straight ahead in order to keep your back straight. Pull your elbow up as high as possible without twisting your torso. Avoid jerking the weight upward.

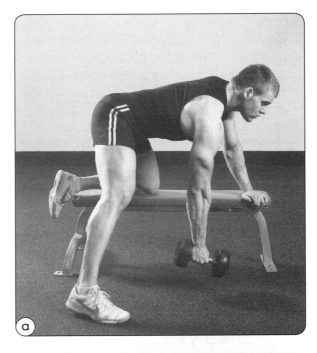

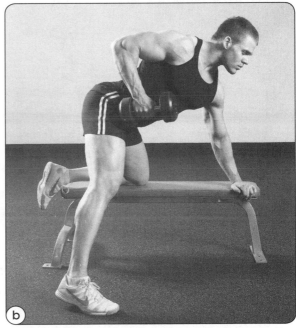

Figure 14.9 Dumbbell row: *(a)* Grip the dumbbell in one hand; *(b)* lift the weight straight upward.

Lumbar Extension

Position yourself facedown across the lumbar extension apparatus, with your hips supported on the bench and your heels secured under the ankle pads. Bend forward at the waist so that your torso hangs down toward the floor. Cross your arms in front of your chest (figure 14.10*a*). In the start position, your torso should be perpendicular at 90 degrees to your thighs. Begin the exercise by lifting your body at the waist. Straighten all the way up until your torso is slightly above parallel to the ground (figure 14.10*b*). The angle of your spine should change from being curled forward to arched slightly backward at full extension. Despite the name of this exercise, do not hyperextend your lower back because this places excess pressure on the joints of your spine. Momentarily hold the extended position just above parallel before slowly returning to the start position.

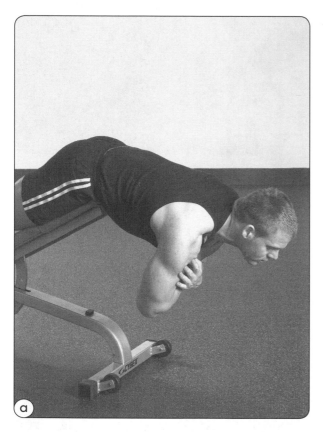 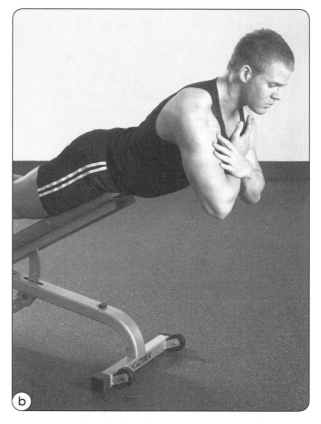

Figure 14.10 Lumbar extension: *(a)* Lie over an extension bench; *(b)* lift your torso to just beyond parallel.

▶ **CHECK IT!** To make the lower back work harder, hold a weight plate across the front of your chest.

You can make this exercise less strenuous by using an incline extension bench. The ankle support is lower to the ground, and your legs make a 45-degree angle to the floor.

Preacher Curl

Sit facing a preacher bench with the pad touching your lower chest. The pad should slope away from the front of your body at about 45 degrees. Grab a dumbbell in one hand, and rest the back of your upper arm on the pad. The pad should support your arm from the armpit to the elbow. In the start position, your arm is out straight with your palm turned up (figure 14.11*a*). Begin the repetition by bending your elbow, curling the dumbbell up until it reaches shoulder level (figure 14.11*b*). Pause at the top for a second, contracting the biceps. Slowly lower the weight. Stop 10 degrees short of full elbow extension to keep tension on the biceps at the bottom of the lift. Hold the weight for one second and repeat. The preacher bench isolates the biceps muscle because movement can occur only at the elbow. At the completion of the set, switch hands and perform the same movement with the other arm.

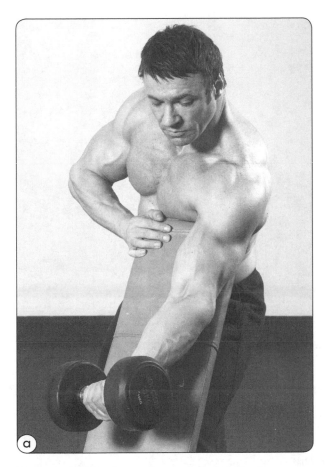 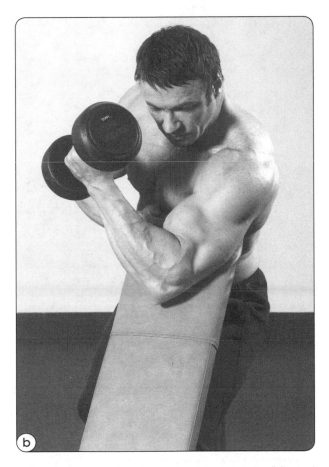

Figure 14.11 Preacher curl: *(a)* Rest arm on preacher bench with dumbbell in hand; *(b)* curl dumbbell to shoulder.

▶ **CHECK IT!** Stopping short of full elbow extension as you lower the weight keeps tension on the biceps and reduces the risk of tendon injury.

As an alternative, you can also perform preacher curls using a barbell or a biceps curl machine with a sloping armrest. You can also perform the same exercise using an incline bench.

Concentration Curl

Grab a dumbbell and sit on the edge of a flat bench. Rest the back of your upper arm against the inside of your thigh. In the start position, your arm is straight and your palm turned up (figure 14.12*a*). Lift the dumbbell toward your shoulder (figure 14.12*b*). Keep your upper arm and torso still; let your biceps do the work. When the dumbbell reaches shoulder level, pause for one second, then slowly lower the weight. Stop a few degrees short of full extension to keep tension on your biceps. Pause momentarily and repeat. When you have completed the set, switch the dumbbell to your other hand to work the opposite biceps.

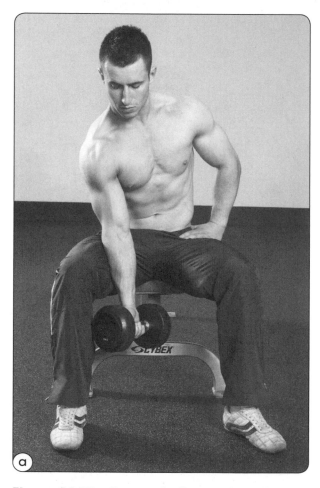 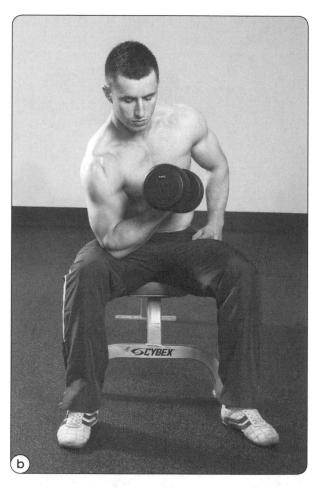

Figure 14.12   Concentration curl: *(a)* Sit on a flat bench with a dumbbell in one hand; *(b)* curl the dumbbell toward your shoulder.

▶ **CHECK IT!**   Keep your upper arm and torso still; let your biceps do the work.

You can also do this exercise using a D handle attached to the cable of a low pulley.

Barbell Wrist Curl

Sit on an exercise bench. Grab a barbell in a shoulder-width underhand grip, palms turned up. Position the back of your forearms on the tops of your thighs so that your wrists extend beyond your knees (figure 14.13*a*). Or you can rest your forearms on the bench between your thighs. Lower the weight slowly by bending your wrists toward the floor (figure 14.13*b*). Feel the muscles of your forearm stretch and hold in the bottom position momentarily. Curl the weight up using wrist motion. Your elbows should not move, and the backs of your forearms should remain in contact with your thighs. Hold the contracted position for one second, then slowly lower the weight and repeat. In the ideal position for this exercise, your forearms make a 45-degree angle to the floor. Try resting your forearms on a preacher bench to see if this works better for you.

▶ **CHECK IT!** Typically this exercise is better performed using a thumbless grip, with your thumbs positioned underneath the bar.

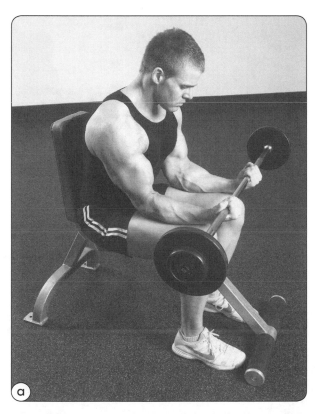 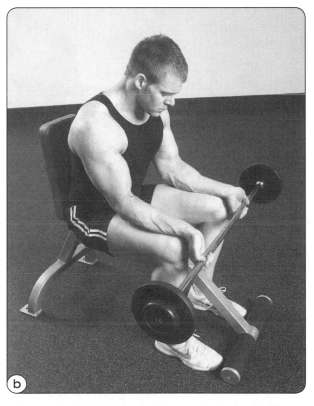

Figure 14.13 Barbell wrist curl: *(a)* Hold the barbell so that your wrists hang over your knees; *(b)* lower the weight by bending your wrists.

Reverse Wrist Curl

As the name suggests, the reverse wrist curl is identical to the standard wrist curl except you take a reverse overhand grip on the bar, palms turned down. This exercise works the muscles on the backside of your forearm. The fronts of your forearms rest on your thighs or the bench so that your hands are hanging off the edge (figure 14.14*a*). Slowly lower the weight by bending your wrists toward the floor (figure 14.14*b*). Feel the muscles stretch; hold for one count. Curl the weight up, moving the back of your hands toward you. Motion should occur at the wrist, not the elbow. Your forearms remain in contact with your thighs or the bench. Hold the contracted position for one second, then slowly lower the weight and repeat. You can do this exercise using a preacher bench or with a dumbbell in each hand in place of the barbell.

▶ **CHECK IT!** In contrast to the standard wrist curl, the reverse wrist curl is best performed using a normal grip with your thumbs curled around the bar.

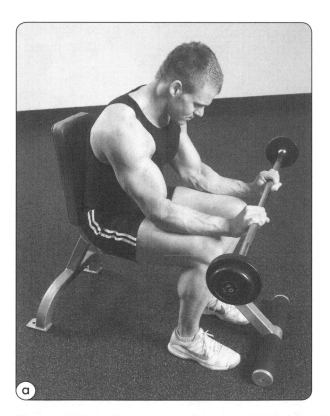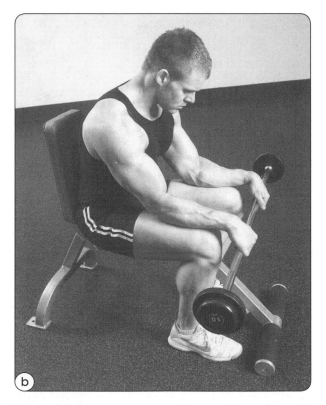

Figure 14.14 Reverse wrist curl: *(a)* Hold the barbell so your wrists hang over your knees; *(b)* lower the weight by bending your wrists.

Cardio (Wednesday)

Perform 30 minutes of aerobic exercise. Choose from cycling, walking, jogging, stair climbing, using an elliptical cross-trainer, or jumping rope.

Legs (Thursday)

QUADRICEPS

Leg Extension

Sit at a leg extension machine. Adjust the backrest so that the backs of your knees fit snugly against the seat and your thighs are supported. Position your ankles under the roller pad. If the pad is adjustable, position it so it rests just above your ankles on the lowest part of your shins. Grip the handles on the sides of the machine for support (figure 14.15a). From the start position, contract your quadriceps to straighten your knees (figure 14.15b). Lift the weight all the way up until your knees are straight. Pause for one second at the top and flex your quadriceps. Slowly lower the weight until your knees are bent to 90 degrees. Hold the weight momentarily in the bottom position and then repeat.

▶ **CHECK IT!**   Do not let your hips rise off the seat. Avoid bending your knees beyond 90 degrees, as this will cause stress on the knee joint.

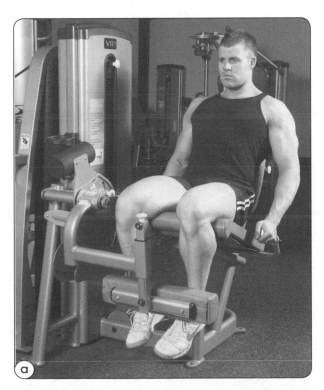 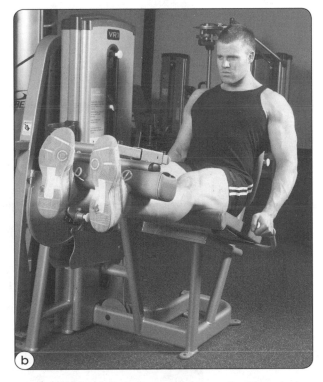

Figure 14.15   Leg extension: *(a)* Get into position in a leg extension machine; *(b)* straighten your legs.

Leg Press

Get into position on the seat of a leg press machine. Place your feet about shoulder-width apart on the foot plate, toes pointing out slightly. In the start position, your legs should be fully straight with knees locked (figure 14.16a). Before you begin, use the handle to release the weight support. Slowly lower the weight until your knees bend to 90 degrees (figure 14.16b). At this point, your thighs should lightly touch your abdomen. Inhale deeply as the weight is lowered. Push the weight back to the start position by straightening your knees. Exhale as you lift the weight. If you want to keep tension on the quadriceps, don't quite lock out your knees at the top.

▶ **CHECK IT!** The backrest should be at a 45- to 60-degree angle to the seat. When the angle is closer to 90 degrees, excessive strain is placed on your lower spine.

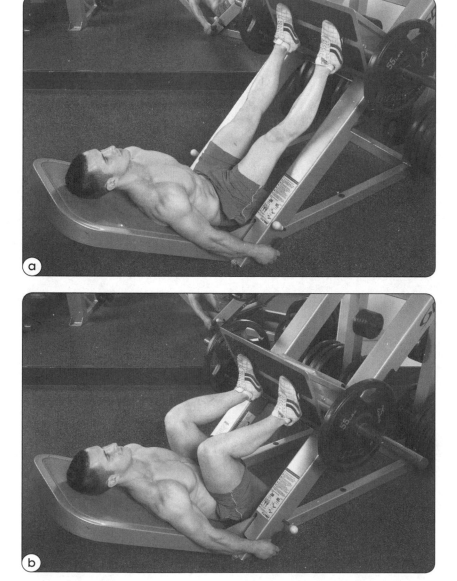

Figure 14.16 Leg press: (a) Sit in a leg press machine with legs straight; (b) lower the weight by bending your knees.

QUADRICEPS

Machine Squat

Use a Smith machine if one is available. Position the bar of the machine centrally across the upper portion of your back. Stand with your feet shoulder-width apart slightly in front of the plane of your body, toes pointing forward (figure 14.17a). This is the start position. Begin the repetition by bending your knees and slowly lowering your hips straight down until your thighs are parallel to the floor (figure 14.17b). During the movement, keep your back straight, your chin up, and your head looking forward. Once you reach the bottom position, push the weight up using your thighs and hips until your knees are straight. On a Smith machine, the movement occurs in a single plane vertically up and down perpendicular to the floor. Inhale deeply during the descent, and exhale on the way up.

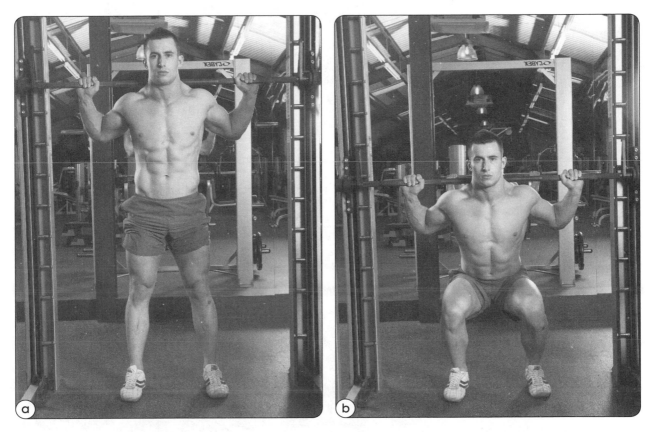

Figure 14.17 Machine squat: (a) Get into position in the machine; (b) lower the weight by bending your knees.

▶ **CHECK IT!** To reduce the chance of knee injury, avoid squatting below parallel. Position your feet about six inches (15 cm) in front of the plane of your body during machine squats to optimize trajectory.

A good alternative to Smith machine squats would be to utilize the hack-squat machine with your shoulders under the pads and your spine supported against the back rest. If you don't have access to a Smith machine or hack-squat machine, you may perform standard barbell squats, as described in chapter 7.

Leg Curl

Position yourself on a leg curl machine, and place the backs of your ankles on the roller pads (figure 14.18a). Grip the handles for support. From the start position, curl the weight up by bending your knees (figure 14.18b). Bring your heels toward your buttocks. Hold the contracted position for one second. Slowly return the weight to the start position until your legs are almost straight. Hold momentarily and then repeat.

You can also do this exercise using a lying leg curl machine.

▶ **CHECK IT!** Don't lift your hips off the machine. Stop a few degrees short of full knee extension to keep tension on the hamstrings.

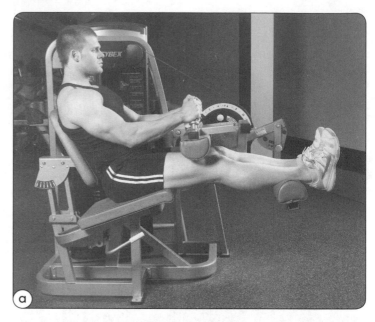

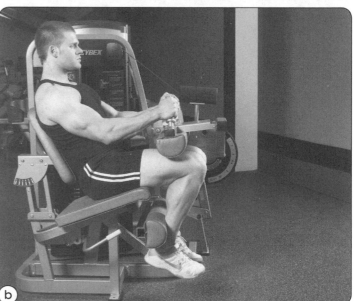

Figure 14.18 Leg curl: *(a)* Get into position on the leg curl machine; *(b)* curl the weight toward your buttocks.

HAMSTRINGS

Straight-Leg Deadlift

Pick up a barbell in an overhand grip (palms down) with your hands shoulder-width apart. Stand straight, holding the barbell at arms' length in front of you. Place your feet directly below your hips, toes pointing forward (figure 14.19*a*). From the start position, bend forward at the hips, slowly lowering the barbell vertically downward (figure 14.19*b*). Don't bend at the knees. Keep your back straight and your chin up. Descend until the weight passes below knee level and you feel your hamstring muscles stretch. Do not allow the weight to touch the floor. At the bottom, contract your hamstrings and gluteus muscles to lift the weight back to the start position.

▶ **CHECK IT!** Do not hunch your back. If your hamstrings are tight, you can allow a slight bend at the knees, but no more than about 20 degrees.

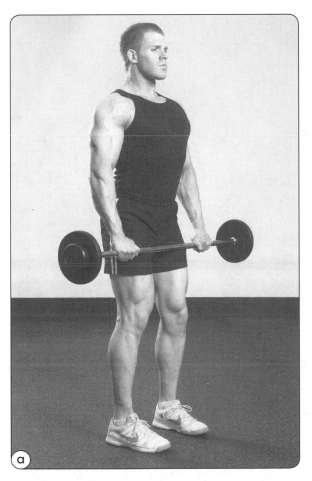 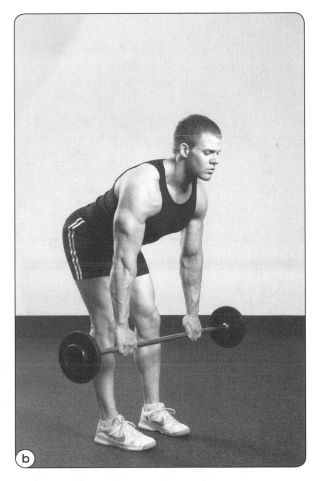

Figure 14.19 Straight-leg deadlift: *(a)* Hold the barbell at arms' length; *(b)* lower the weight, keeping your knees locked.

CALVES

Seated Calf Raise

Position yourself on a seated calf machine. Place the balls of your feet on the platform and the knee pad on the front of your lower thighs. Your knees should be in line with your hips, with your toes directly below your knees (figure 14.20*a*). Release the safety catch and grip the handles. Slowly lower your heels as far as you can, stretching your calf muscles but keeping your toes firmly on the platform (figure 14.20*b*). In the bottom position, hold the stretch for one second. Contract your calf muscles and push the weight as high as possible, as if you were standing on tiptoes. Flex hard at the top and hold for another single count. Slowly lower the weight and repeat.

▶ **CHECK IT!** Don't rest the pad too high on your thigh. It should be placed just above your knees.

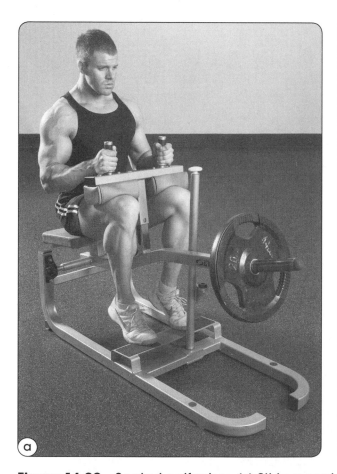 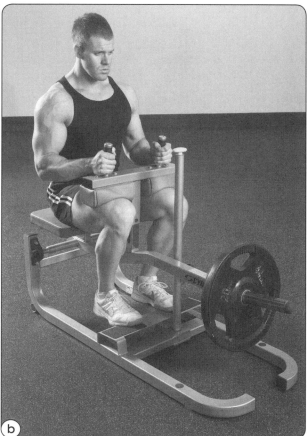

Figure 14.20 Seated calf raise: *(a)* Sit in a seated calf machine; *(b)* lower your heels.

Straight-Leg Calf Raise

Get into position on the seat of a leg press machine. Place the balls of both feet on the lower edge of the foot plate, about six inches (15 cm) apart, toes pointing forward. Make sure your heels are free to move beneath the foot plate. Lock your knees out straight so that motion occurs exclusively at the ankles (figure 14.21*a*). From the start position, push the weight up as far as you can. Hold the tiptoes position momentarily as you contract your calf muscles (figure 14.21*b*). Slowly lower the weight back to the start position. In the bottom position, pause to stretch the calf muscles, then repeat. Several machines are designed for performing straight-leg calf raises in a seated position with support for the lumbar spine. If you don't have access to a leg press or calf sled machine, perform standing calf raises (chapter 7) or donkey calf raises (chapter 10).

▶ **CHECK IT!** Keep your knees stiff throughout the movement.

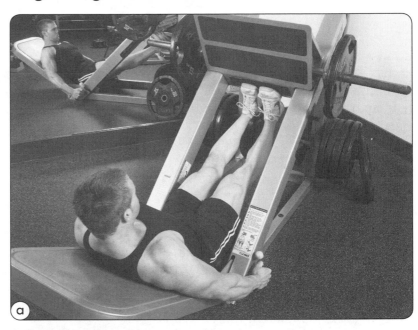

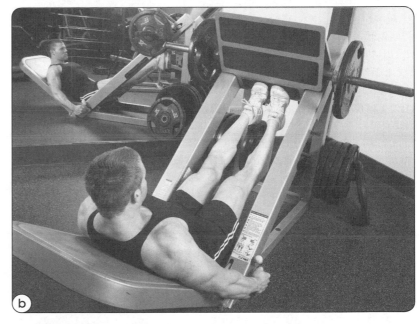

Figure 14.21 Straight-leg calf raise: *(a)* Position your feet on the foot plate; *(b)* push the weight upward, pointing your toes.

ROTATOR CUFF

External Rotation

External rotations build the infraspinatus and teres minor muscles that lie behind the shoulder under the rear deltoid. Adjust the cable pulley to waist height. Stand with the left side of your body beside the weight stack. Grab the cable handle with your right hand, palm turned toward the pulley (figure 14.22*a*). Position your right elbow firmly against your waist, elbow bent at 90 degrees and forearm parallel to the floor. Begin with the handle at the midline of your body, and move your hand toward your right side as far as it will go (figure 14.22*b*). Be sure to stand far enough away from the pulley so that the cable remains under tension. Keep your elbow fixed at your side and your forearm parallel to the floor throughout the movement. Your hand should move through an arc of approximately 90 degrees. Hold the contracted position momentarily before slowly returning to the start position. After completing the set, switch positions and perform with the left hand.

> **CHECK IT!** Only the hand and forearm move during this exercise. Keep the elbow and upper arm tight against the side of your body. From your viewpoint, the motion resembles the hand of a clock moving back and forth between 10 o'clock and 2 o'clock.

You can also do this exercise by tying one end of a rubber exercise band around a fixed upright support at waist height.

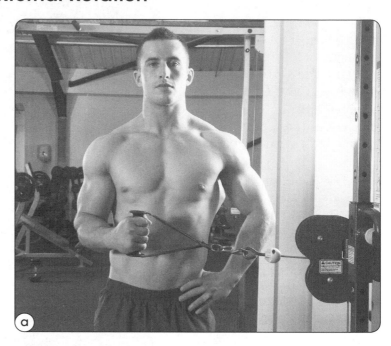

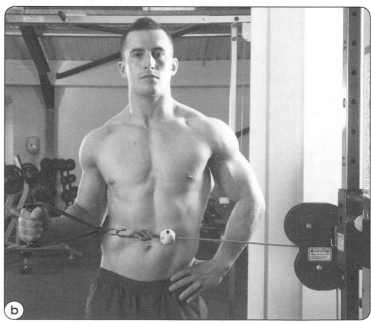

Figure 14.22 External rotation: *(a)* Start with the handle at the middle of your body; *(b)* pull handle outward to the right.

Internal Rotation

Internal rotations build the subscapularis muscle that lies under the front deltoid. Adjust the cable pulley to waist height. Stand with the left side of your body beside the weight stack. Grab the cable handle with your left hand, palm turned away from the pulley (figure 14.23*a*). Position your left elbow firmly against your waist, elbow bent at 90 degrees and forearm parallel to the floor. With the handle out to the side, pull the cable inward across the front of your body (figure 14.23*b*). Keep your elbow fixed at your side and your forearm parallel to the floor at all times. Hold the contracted position momentarily, then return slowly to the start position. Be sure to stand far enough away from the pulley so that the cable remains under tension throughout. Your hand should move through an arc of about 90 to 120 degrees. When the set is complete, switch positions and perform with the right hand.

▶ **CHECK IT!** Only the hand and forearm move during this exercise. Keep the elbow and upper arm tight against the side of your body. The motion resembles the hand of a clock moving back and forth between 10 o'clock and 2 o'clock.

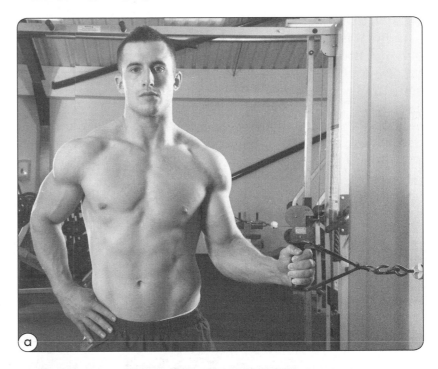

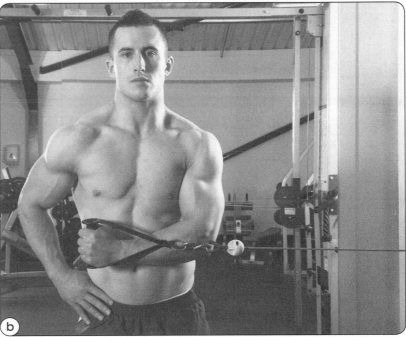

Figure 14.23 Internal rotation: *(a)* Grab the handle out to your side; *(b)* pull the handle across your body.

Cable Lateral Raise (Abduction)

This exercise strengthens the supraspinatus muscle, which lies over the top of the shoulder. The movement is similar to the dumbbell lateral raise for the deltoid (chapter 7). Position the cable pulley at floor level. Stand with your left side next to the weight stack. Grasp the handle attached to the low pulley, with your right hand crossed over your body (figure 14.24*a*). Raise your hand up and out in a wide arc (figure 14.24*b*). Keep your hand slightly in front of the plane of your body. Keep your elbow fairly straight; the elbow joint should not bend during the movement. Raise your hand to shoulder level, hold momentarily, then slowly lower the weight to the start position. After completing the set, switch positions and face the opposite direction. Repeat the exercise with your left hand.

▶ **CHECK IT!** The supraspinatus muscle is worked best during the first 60 degrees of this motion, so there's no need to raise your hand above shoulder level.

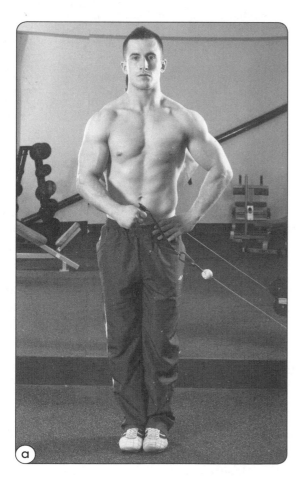 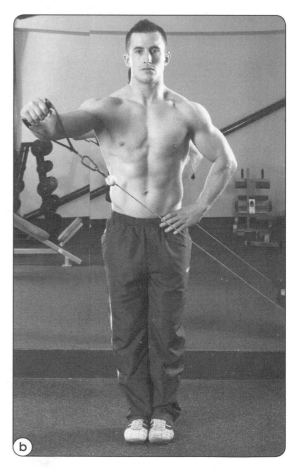

Figure 14.24 Cable lateral raise: *(a)* Grab the handle on the low pulley; *(b)* raise your hand in a wide arc.

DELTOIDS

Machine Upright Row

Position the cable pulley at floor level. Stand facing away from the weight stack. Using an overhand grip, grasp the short bar attached to the low pulley, with the cable passing between your legs (figure 14.25*a*). From the start position, raise your elbows outward and upward from the side of your body until your upper arms are parallel to the floor (figure 14.25*b*). Pause momentarily when your elbows reach shoulder level, and contract the deltoid muscles forcibly. Slowly lower your elbows back to the start position and repeat. Keep your back straight throughout the movement. Think of your hands as hooks. Lift the elbows, keeping your forearms vertical and perpendicular to the floor.

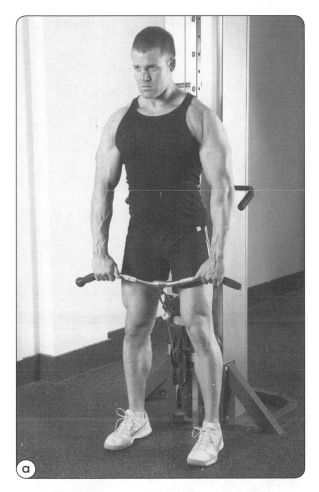 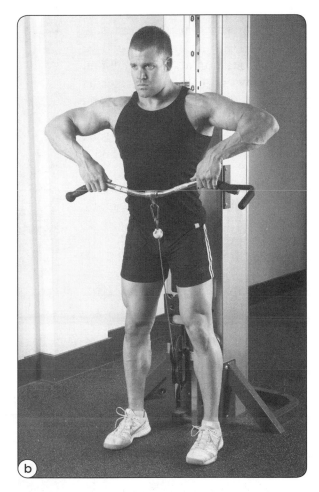

Figure 14.25 Machine upright row: *(a)* Grab the bar; *(b)* raise elbows upward.

▶ **CHECK IT!** Don't raise your elbows too high as this places unnecessary stress on the shoulder joints and risks injury to the rotator cuff.

You can also do this exercise using a Smith machine. If you don't have access to machines, do this exercise using a barbell.

Rear Deltoid Fly

Sit facing the deltoid fly machine, with your chest against the pad. Adjust the seat height so your arms are parallel to the floor when you grasp the handles (figure 14.26a). From the start position, slowly pull the handles back until your arms make a straight line across your body. Hold for one second, contracting the rear deltoid muscle (figure 14.26b). Slowly return to the start position and repeat. Keep your elbows slightly bent with arms parallel to the floor throughout the movement. This exercise works the rear portion of the deltoid muscle, which overlies the back of the shoulder.

If you do not have access to a rear deltoid machine or reverse chest fly machine, this exercise can be performed using dumbbells with your torso bent forward at the waist.

▶ **CHECK IT!** Adjust the seat height so that when you grasp the handles, your hands are level with your shoulders and your arms are parallel to the floor. To isolate the rear deltoids, grasp the horizontal handles (if available) with a palms-down grip.

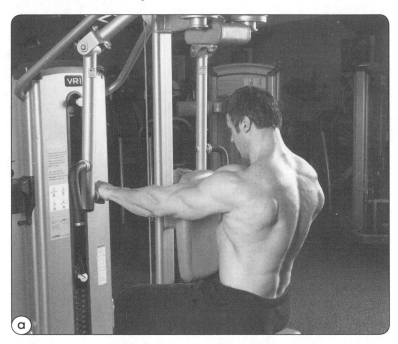

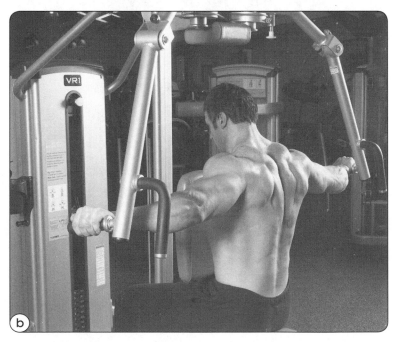

Figure 14.26 Rear deltoid fly: (a) Sit facing the machine and grasp the handles; (b) pull your hands back in an arc.

Front Deltoid Raise

Grab a dumbbell by interlocking the fingers of both hands around the bar. Let your arms hang straight down in front of you. Hold the dumbbell vertically, with the uppermost weight resting against your thumbs (figure 14.27a). From this start position, perform a front raise by lifting the dumbbell up in front of you. The motion occurs exclusively at the shoulder; keep your elbows nearly straight. Stop the raise when your arms are parallel to the floor (figure 14.27b). Hold this position momentarily, squeezing a contraction in your front deltoids. Lower the weight slowly down to the start position, and then repeat.

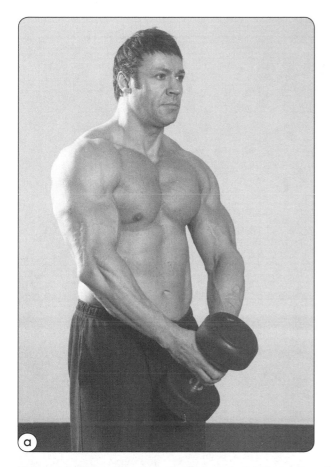 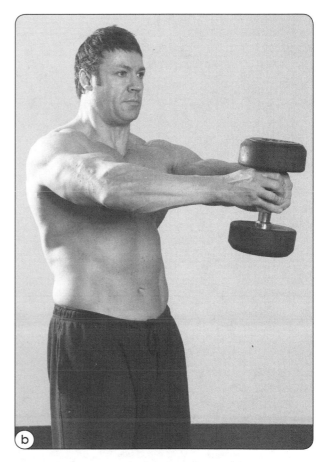

Figure 14.27 Front deltoid raise: *(a)* Hold the dumbbell at arms' length; *(b)* raise the dumbbell forward.

▶ **CHECK IT!** Holding the dumbbell is easier if you rest the inside of the upper end against your interlocked thumbs and index fingers.

You can also do this exercise with a dumbbell in each hand. Raise one dumbbell at a time, working the right and left deltoids alternately.

Shrug

Shrugs build the trapezius muscles in the space between your neck and shoulder. The traps also pass down behind your neck, forming the central portion of your upper back. To perform shrugs, stand upright with a dumbbell in each hand, hands hanging at your sides (figure 14.28*a*). With your palms turned in, shrug your shoulders as high as you can (figure 14.28*b*). Try to touch your ears with the tops of both shoulders. Hold the contracted position for one second. Slowly lower the weights, stretching your traps in the bottom position. Hold for one count and repeat. Restrict motion to your shoulder girdle; don't bend your elbows. Move the weight vertically up and down about six inches (15 cm).

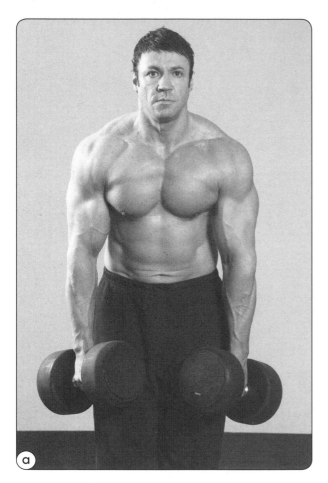 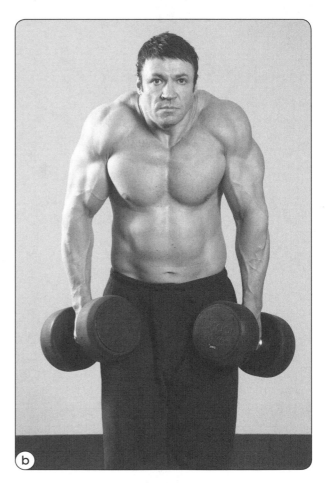

Figure 14.28 Shrug: *(a)* Stand with dumbbells in hand; *(b)* bring your shoulders toward your ears.

▶ **CHECK IT!** Look straight ahead, and keep your back erect.

You can also do this exercise using a barbell held at arms' length in front with palms turned toward you. Personally, I prefer machine shrugs.

Machine Crunch

Sit on the seat of an abdominal crunch machine. Depending on the machine design, the resistance may be transmitted via handles or pads. Position your feet on the floor, or on a footrest (figure 14.29a). From the start position, crunch forward and down with your abdominal muscles, curling your torso toward your knees. Hold momentarily in the crunch position, forcibly contracting your abs (figure 14.29b). Then slowly return to the start position and repeat.

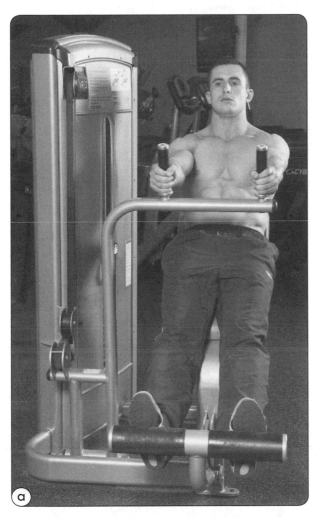 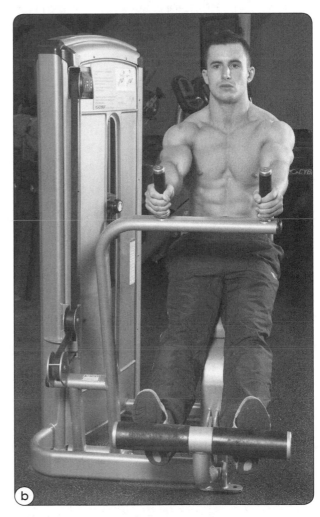

Figure 14.29 Machine crunch: *(a)* Sit in the seat of the ab machine; *(b)* crunch your torso forward and downward.

▶ **CHECK IT!** Do not go back too far, as this will release tension from the abs and place undue stress on the lower back.

If you don't have access to an abdominal crunch machine, you could do floor crunches (chapter 10) or decline sit-ups (chapter 7) to work your upper abdominal muscles.

Bench Leg Raise

Sit on the edge of a flat exercise bench. Grip the bench behind you. With knees slightly bent, allow your legs to hang down, heels almost touching the floor. Lean back until your torso makes a 45-degree angle to the bench. Support yourself with your hands (figure 14.30a). Begin the exercise by pulling your thighs toward your chest, keeping your legs together (figure 14.30b). Tighten your lower abs as your hips bend up. Stop before your thighs become vertical, and hold the contracted position for one second. Slowly lower your legs. Stop before your heels make contact with the ground. Hold in the bottom position for a single count and repeat. This is a terrific exercise for the lower abs.

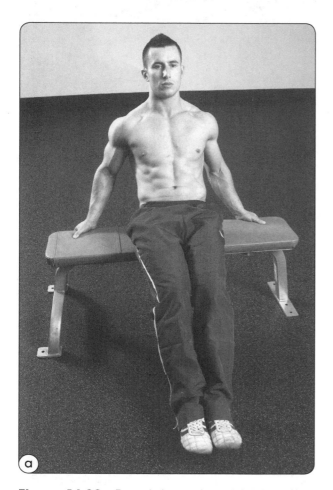 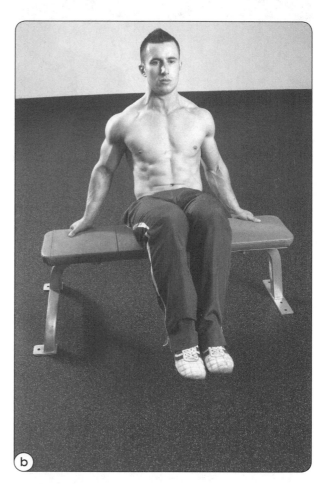

Figure 14.30 Bench leg raise: *(a)* Sit on the bench; *(b)* pull your thighs to your chest.

▶ **CHECK IT!** Lower your legs slowly to keep tension on your abs.

Alternative versions of the leg raise exercise include the incline leg raise (chapter 7) and the vertical leg raise (chapter 10). Personal preference will decide which version of the exercise works best for you.

Cardio (Saturday)

Perform 30 minutes of aerobic exercise. Choose from cycling, walking, jogging, stair climbing, using an elliptical cross-trainer, or jumping rope.

PART V

Muscle Maintenance

In part V, you'll discover how to maintain and care for your muscles with my top tips for body-sculpting longevity. Chapter 15 reveals the trade secrets for fixing faults in your physique. Do you want to know how to get that teardrop muscle in your thigh or how to target your rear deltoid? Discover how to fix physique symmetry, improve proportion, and get that athletic V-shape taper. In chapter 16, you'll get the doctor's prescription for muscle care, including tips for treating and preventing injury. Chapter 17 reveals survival strategies for the peak physique, skills that make muscle maintenance easy. You'll learn how to prevent pitfalls in your progress and burst out of any training plateau.

Advanced Sculpting Solutions and Training Tips

In this chapter you'll discover a selection of advanced technical tricks to modify exercises for maximum effect. I'll show you my blueprint for creating an advanced body-sculpting workout. Small technical adjustments can make a world of difference—tricks you've never even thought of, like changing your grip, spacing your hands, adjusting your stance, positioning your feet, varying the trajectory of the lift, or manipulating the start and finish positions of the exercise. Make no mistake, this chapter will help take your training to a more advanced level. You'll learn how to achieve a pump in those hard-to-hit spots such as the rear deltoid, triceps horseshoe, and quadriceps teardrop. You'll also discover how to target areas of special needs, fixing asymmetry, fine-tuning your V-shape taper, improving vascularity, and achieving that extra-lean look.

If you want to modify any exercise for maximum effect, there are several options you can consider—think of it as a body-sculpting blueprint. The technical considerations for your blueprint should include grip, range of motion, hand spacing, trajectory, isolation, variation, foot positioning, and stance. Now let's see how these factors can be incorporated to advance your workouts.

DELTOIDS

Anytime you change hand position or grip, you make a technical adjustment that changes the biomechanics of the exercise. Making such modifications targets different areas of a muscle. For shoulders, the front raise is one of the best exercises to isolate the front deltoid. When you use a barbell, your hands are fixed in a *pronated* grip, with your palms facing downward. This grip places the shoulder joint in a position of internal rotation that allows the lateral deltoid to assist in the exercise. The same applies when you perform dumbbell front raises with a palms-down pronated grip. However, if you switch dumbbell position to a *neutral* grip with your thumbs pointing upward and palms facing together, the shoulder joint is externally rotated. This position minimizes lateral deltoid assistance, focusing all the effort on the anterior deltoid. So, holding the dumbbells with a neutral thumbs-up grip is the best way to target your anterior deltoid.

The rear deltoid fly is an excellent exercise for targeting the rear deltoid, and the movement will work the rear deltoid effectively whether your grab the vertical or the horizontal handles. However, there is a subtle difference between the two hand positions. When you grab the handles with your hands vertical (thumbs upward, palms facing together), the shoulder joint is in a position of neutral rotation. This allows the lateral deltoid to participate in the movement, so you are working both the lateral and rear portions of the deltoid with your hands in this position. When your hands are in the horizontal position (palms down, thumbs facing together),

Behind-the-Neck Barbell Press: Is it a good or bad exercise?

The behind-the-neck barbell press is touted as one of the best exercises to add mass to your deltoids, but it carries a significant risk of shoulder injury. Believe me, as an orthopedic surgeon, I know a thing or two about shoulder injuries, and in my opinion, the behind-the-neck barbell press is a biomechanical time bomb. Let me elaborate.

The shoulder is the most mobile joint in your body. It allows you to windmill your arm through 360 degrees of motion. But this mechanical freedom comes with a price—vulnerability. You see, the shoulder joint sacrifices *stability* for *mobility*. The head of the upper arm bone sits in a small shallow socket, much like a golf ball balances precariously on a golf tee. Your shoulder joint is not designed to perform activities behind the plane of your body. Combing your hair, scratching your back, and dealing with toilet hygiene are acceptable activities. But lifting weights behind your head or back is a fast track to shoulder injury.

The behind-the-neck barbell press is bad news. In my opinion, it's probably one of the most dangerous shoulder exercises, even if executed with perfect form. The exercise places the shoulder in extreme abduction and external rotation (the high-five position), where the shoulder is most vulnerable to injury. This exercise can cause shoulder instability, rotator cuff damage, and neck injury. And these risks far outweigh any bodybuilding benefits.

You might be able to get away with behind-the-neck barbell presses when you are young. But as the years go by, this movement will slowly grind away at your rotator cuff, resulting in chronic shoulder pain or a torn muscle. There are no specific advantages to this movement that can't be achieved with other safer exercises. If you want pain-free shoulders and longevity in the gym, my advice is to choose a safe shoulder workout and avoid behind-the-neck presses.

the shoulder is internally rotated. And this subtle change places the lateral head at a mechanical disadvantage, which makes the rear deltoid work harder. So in effect, the horizontal hand position is superior if you really want to isolate the rear deltoid. This effect also applies to bent-over dumbbell raises. Raising the dumbbells with your palms facing together works both the lateral and rear deltoid muscles. But if you hold the dumbbells using a pronated grip with your thumbs pointing inward, your shoulders are in a position of internal rotation, and your rear deltoids will be better isolated.

BICEPS

In general, the biceps muscle tends to respond better to a short, heavy workout with a few key exercises rather than an hour-long dance around every biceps station in the gym. Instead of giving you the same old advice for a generic biceps routine that you can find in any bodybuilding publication, I'm going to give you some technical suggestions to improve your biceps workouts.

- **Grip.** Performing curls using a dumbbell allows you to work the biceps through two motions, namely elbow flexion and hand supination. When using a straight bar, hands are fixed in full supination (palms up), which helps maximize biceps contraction as the elbow is flexed. When using an EZ bar, the grip switches from the fully supinated position into a less supinated, nearly neutral grip (palms facing in). This hand position is less strenuous on the wrist joints and tends to focus effort on the outer (long) head of the biceps and the brachialis muscle.
- **Range of motion.** Stopping a few degrees short of full elbow extension keeps tension on the biceps as the weight is lowered.
- **Hand spacing.** A wide grip on the bar focuses effort on the inner biceps (short head), whereas a narrow grip works the outer biceps (long head).
- **Trajectory.** The position of the upper arm (relative to the floor) changes the focus of effort. When the arm is vertical (shoulder directly above the elbow), resistance increases as the weight is raised, and effort is focused on the upper biceps (peak). With the arm at an inclined angle (elbow in front of the shoulder), resistance is maximal at the start, so effort is targeted on the lower section of the biceps at the elbow.
- **Isolation.** Fixing the upper arm (e.g., on the preacher bench) prevents movement at the shoulder and is an excellent way to isolate the biceps. What's more, performing curls one arm at time, whether using a dumbbell, cable, or machine, helps focus your effort.
- **Variation.** Different exercises provide a different stimulus. Try switching exercises each week or every month to keep the muscle "guessing." Alternating between barbells, dumbbells, machines, and cables will hit the muscle in different ways.

TRICEPS

Fixing faults in your physique is an ongoing challenge for any serious bodybuilder. Whether it's adding mass, losing fat, or improving proportion or symmetry, your body sculpture is a work in progress. As you've already discovered, targeting subsections of the triceps is not that easy. Even though the muscle has three sections, the triceps has only one primary action, to straighten the elbow. During most triceps exercises, the inner portion does most of the work because it is the largest component of the muscle. However, you can incorporate subtle modifications into your triceps workout to help target the outer muscle belly.

There are two biomechanical adjustments that force the outer triceps to contribute more effort during an exercise. The first trick is to pronate your hand so that the palm faces downward. Pronation is the opposing movement to supination. To distinguish between these two motions, think of a money transaction. When you give change, your hand is pronated, but when you receive change, your hand is supinated. Give change, get change. Got it? Forcibly pronating your hand during a triceps exercise will target the outer portion of the muscle. A good exercise for this is cable triceps push-down using a rope attachment. As you straighten the elbow, pronate your hands in an outward direction.

The second trick is to internally rotate your shoulder and arm. For example, when triceps dips are performed in a standard fashion, your palms face each other with your thumbs pointing forward. Well, try doing dips (or machine dips) with your arms rotated inward so that your grip is flipped, with your palms facing outward and thumbs pointing back.

Another way to target the outer triceps is to preexhaust the inner muscle with a traditional mass builder such as dips or close-grip bench presses. Then with the inner head burned out, move quickly to an isolation exercise such as one-arm cable push-downs with the D handle. Use an overhand grip so that your hand is pronated. The outer head is forced to work because the inner head is exhausted from the previous exercise. You can feel the outer head contracting with your free hand. Try these techniques during your next triceps workout, and very soon you'll be the owner of a pair of lucky horseshoes!

FOREARMS

Unlike the front of the upper arm, where size is largely attributable to one muscle (the biceps), the flexor aspect of the forearm contains no fewer than nine different muscles. Six forearm muscles participate in the standard wrist curl exercise. Three of these muscles flex the wrist joint, and the other three muscles flex the digits (as when you make a fist or grip a bar).

Weak Wrists: My wrists hurt when I lift heavy; what can I do?

Wrist pain is often caused by a compressive load across the joint, typically inflicted during pressing movements. Correct technique is key here. Make sure you keep your wrist stiff and straight, with your knuckles in line with your forearm. Avoid cocking your wrist back or angling it to the side. You could also be proactive in preventing this problem by strengthening your forearm muscles using wrist curls. If all else fails, you might consider using some wrist supports.

When you apply this basic anatomic knowledge, it becomes apparent that the finger muscles make a significant contribution to forearm size. So, if you want to maximize the amount of meat in your forearms, you'd be wise to incorporate a movement that directly works the finger flexor muscles. With this in mind, the standard wrist curl will be more effective if you allow the bar to roll down along your fingers during the negative phase of the exercise. The early positive phase targets the finger flexors as you finger-curl the bar into your palm. And the late positive phase works the other forearm flexors as you curl the wrist upward.

When I perform wrist curls, I use the full movement initially, allowing the bar to roll down to my fingertips before curling the weight back up. Then, when the finger flexors fatigue, I continue the exercise with a clenched-fist grip on the bar until the wrist flexors reach failure. This technique essentially prefatigues the weaker finger flexors during the full-range first portion of the set before you blast the stronger wrist flexors during the partial-range second half of the set. Using this method, you'll fatigue *all* the flexor muscles of the forearm, and the end result will be more muscle mass. Try this technique during your next forearm workout, and very soon, people will be calling you Popeye (you know, the cartoon character with the humongous forearms?). Oh, and don't forget to exercise the extensor muscles on the backside of your forearm with a suitable exercise such as reverse wrist curls or hammer curls.

GLUTES

The big muscle that gives shape to your butt is the gluteus maximus. It arises from a large area on the rear of the pelvic bone, passes down behind the hip joint, and attaches onto the upper femur. When it contracts, this powerful muscle causes hip extension; it is used during routine daily activities such as walking, running, stair climbing, rising from a seated position, squatting, and lifting. The gluteus muscle is worked during several core leg exercises that require hip flexion and extension, namely squats, deadlifts, lunges, and leg presses. The glutes are not really worked during leg exercises where the hip joint is held stiff (e.g., leg extensions and hamstring curls). To maximize gluteus work, it is important to actively contract your glutes at the finish position by squeezing your thighs backward.

Here's a sample leg workout that places emphasis on the gluteus:

1. Leg extensions: These prefatigue the quads, thereby maximizing gluteus work during the exercises that follow.

2. Barbell squats: Go deep, and contract your butt at the top.

3. Stiff-leg deadlifts: In addition to building hamstrings, this exercise will beef out your butt.

4. Walking lunges: This is a great final exercise to light a furnace in your quads, hams, and glutes.

QUADRICEPS

The quadriceps is the largest muscle group in the body. It is made up of four separate muscles: the vastus medialis, vastus lateralis, vastus intermedius, and rectus femoris. Because all four muscles act together during a quad workout, it's a tough task for many bodybuilders to isolate individual thigh muscles. I've no doubt that you work hard during your leg workouts, and you've probably done squats, leg presses, hack squats, and lunges until you were blue in the face. But that stubborn vastus medialis "teardrop" just won't blossom, right? If you want to tease that teardrop out of its shell, you've got to make use of some strategic biomechanical principles. The best exercise that lends itself to these techniques is the leg extension movement, and here's the scoop.

Switching foot position under the roller pad of the leg extension machine allows you to target different sections of the quadriceps. And with your hands free, you can feel the individual quad muscles to check whether they're contracting hard. When you rotate your feet (like the hands of a clock), the tibia bone of the lower leg rotates, which in turn changes the position of the quad tendon. Pointing your toes inward rotates the quad tendon toward the vastus medialis teardrop, and this slight technical adjustment generates a more focused contraction in the inner section of the quadriceps.

Another biomechanical trick to make the vastus medialis work harder during this exercise is to forcibly adduct your thighs together. One way of achieving this is to place a clenched fist between your knees and attempt to squeeze your thighs together as you perform the leg extension movement. Combining these two techniques of internal rotation and forced adduction demands a certain degree of concentration, and you may have to drop the weight on the machine. Give these techniques a try during your next quad workout, and I guarantee your teardrops will be steamed to perfection!

ASYMMETRY

Side-to-side differences resulting from asymmetric muscular development are common among novice bodybuilders. You see, your dominant arm is about 30 percent stronger than your nondominant arm. So when you first start working out and learning new exercise techniques, the tendency is to favor your dominant side. During an upper body barbell workout, your dominant side will bear more weight and thereby work harder than the nondominant side. The result of this subconscious preference is that the dominant side of your body will grow more quickly during your first few months at the gym. However, as you gain experience in the gym, smaller, weaker muscles will catch up and balance out with time. If you are truly having a tough time improving muscle symmetry, you're going to have to restructure your workouts in order to make the lagging muscle groups work harder. Probably the best way to fix physique asymmetry is to work one limb at a time with unilateral exercises using dumbbells, cables, or machines. You can force one side of your body to work harder by incorporating exercises such as one-arm dumbbell curls, one-arm triceps push-downs, one-arm cable lateral raises, one-arm machine chest flys, one-arm dumbbell rows, one-leg quad extensions, one-leg hamstring curls, or one-leg calf raises. Get the idea? By exercising one limb at a time, you can focus on the lagging muscle group and build it up to match the larger, stronger side. See the special element on unilateral training on page 100 for more information.

V-SHAPE TAPER

That athletic V-shape taper is a sought-after look in body sculpting. The taper appearance is the result of having wide shoulders and a slim waist. Structurally, having long collarbones and narrow hip bones creates the effect. Unfortunately, the shape of your skeleton is genetic, and you can't change its structure. If you are not blessed with the best bone structure, what you can do is modify your muscular shape to *create* a V-shape taper. The key areas to work on are your lateral deltoid, outer latissimus dorsi, waist, and outer quadriceps (vastus lateralis). Your workouts should include the following:

- Lateral deltoid raises for shoulder width
- Wide-grip pull-downs or chin-ups for the torso taper
- Abdominal exercises (and diet) to create a narrow waist
- Narrow-stance squats, leg presses, or lunges for the outer quadriceps sweep

PLATEAU

To make progress in bodybuilding, all the basic components—exercise, nutrition, rest, supplements, and so on—must fit together perfectly like the pieces of a jigsaw puzzle. If you're not witnessing positive changes in your physique, you'll need to carefully evaluate your workout regimen and dietary habits. For your exercise program, you should evaluate the amount of weight, the number of reps and sets, exercise selection, rest intervals, workout time, and recovery periods. For your nutrition program, you must consume the correct number of calories from the right food sources and partition the nutrients (protein, carbohydrate, fat) in the ideal ratios.

If you are stuck in a training rut, the first thing you must identify is the exact goal that you're failing to realize: Is it strength, size, or fat loss? It's easier if you focus on fixing one fault at a time. Here are some suggestions that will help increase muscle size and strength.

1. Stick to three or four workouts per week.
2. Incorporate power exercises such as bench presses, deadlifts, squats, rows, barbell curls, and so on.
3. Lift as much weight as you can safely handle for 6 to 10 reps.
4. Try to increase the resistance you lift as often as possible.
5. Hit your training hard, and get out of the gym within an hour—don't waste time in the gym.
6. Be sure to provide sufficient fuel for your workout.
7. Allow ample time for rest and recovery.
8. Forget about cardio if you want to grow.
9. Vary your routine, and switch exercises around every month or so to keep your muscles responding: Change the flat bench press to incline or decline; switch from barbells, to dumbbells, to machines, and so on.
10. Avoid overtraining.

PUMP

The "pump" occurs when an exercised muscle becomes engorged with blood. This physiological response produces a warm, tight, and mildly painful sensation in the muscle. Although a pump is not absolutely essential for muscle growth, it does indicate that a muscle has been worked adequately. Basically, you need to increase the number of reps to pump your muscles full of blood in addition to taking less rest between sets to keep the muscles engorged. Keep your workout time under an hour; exercising beyond this time drains your energy stores, and muscle won't pump when overfatigued. Drinking water during your workout also helps since your body needs to be well hydrated in order to flush blood into those muscles. Make sure you get adequate rest between workouts and maintain a satisfactory carbohydrate intake—you won't get much of a pump if you're carbohydrate depleted.

There are a variety of tricks you can use to improve the muscle pump you experience during exercise.

1. Preexhaust the muscle: Use an isolation exercise before a compound exercise (e.g., flys before bench presses, extensions before squats).
2. Shorten rest intervals: Reduce the time between sets to one minute or less, and proceed quickly from one exercise to the next.
3. Do supersets: Perform two different exercises for the same muscle group, back to back with no rest between.
4. Do drop sets: When you reach failure, reduce the resistance and continue the exercise.
5. Increase the number of repetitions: Perform at least 10 reps per set.

VASCULARITY

In the world of bodybuilding, the term *vascular* refers to the visibility of surface veins under the skin. Physiologically speaking, these subcutaneous veins serve two main purposes: (1) They help blood flow back to the heart, and (2) they assist with the regulation of body temperature. The visibility of these surface veins is affected by a number of factors, such as body fat, body temperature, and blood pressure. When your body fat percentage is more than 12 percent, you won't see many veins because they are covered by fat. You've got to be lean, with a body fat of 10 percent or less, if you want those veins to pop out. When your body is hot during exercise or warm weather, your veins dilate (or bulge) to help you cool down. When you're cold, on the other hand, the veins constrict (or narrow) to conserve body heat. When your blood pressure increases during exercise, the exercise-induced hyperemia (increased blood flow) expands your veins, enhancing their visibility: the so-called pump effect. Here's a list of possible ways to improve your vascularity and get those veins a-popping.

1. Reduce your body fat below 10 percent.
2. Get a pump on at the gym.
3. Drink a glass of red wine.
4. Wear a tight T-shirt for the mild tourniquet effect.
5. Try a nitric oxide stimulator to enhance blood flow and expand veins.
6. A thermodilation spray or lotion containing methyl salicylate can cause veins to dilate for a few hours.

GETTING EXTRA LEAN

As mentioned in chapter 9, the keys to fat loss are the three Cs: cardio, calories, and carbohydrate. If you reach a plateau, or sticking point, in your body fat percentage, here are three possible solutions:

1. Increase your cardio by extending the duration of aerobic exercise to 45 to 60 minutes or adding extra aerobic sessions to your weekly schedule. You could also try high-intensity interval sprint training (see chapter 8) for a more effective fat burn.

2. Reduce your calorie intake by omitting your cheat day, reducing the number of meals you eat, or subtracting 5 to 10 percent increments from your daily total calorie intake.

3. Cut back your carbohydrate by eliminating carbohydrate foods from your last meal of the day or gradually reducing carbohydrate portions so that the nutrient ratio of your diet moves toward 60 percent protein, 30 percent carbohydrate, and 10 percent fat.

Remember that your energy levels fall as you deplete your intake of carbohydrate. It's tough to maintain a diet that contains only 30 percent carbohydrate (around 100 grams per day) for longer than a few weeks. Many competitive bodybuilders practice *decarbing* and *carbing up* during the week before a contest. For the first three days, carbohydrate intake is reduced to 100 grams per day. Then carbohydrate is reintroduced at rates of 200, 300, and 400 grams per day during the lead-up to the show. The process of carbing up restocks glycogen stores in the muscles to make them look full, hard, and defined on contest day. If you really want to drop your body fat percentage quickly, the sample low-carbohydrate diet shown in table 15.1 will burn body fat with extreme prejudice when combined with daily sessions of cardio.

Table 15.1   High-Protein/Low-Carbohydrate Sample Meal Plan

Meal 1	Six egg whites, scrambled Half a grapefruit Calories: 250
Meal 2	Two 6-oz (175 g) cans of tuna with 40 g rice Calories: 450
Meal 3	6-oz (175 g) lean beef with 40 g rice Calories: 350
Meal 4	Protein shake Calories: 250
Meal 5	One 6-oz (175 g) chicken breast Calories: 200
Daily totals (approximate)	Protein: 225 g (60%) Carbohydrate: 112 g (30%) Fat: 16 g (10%) Calories: 1,500

In this chapter we have discussed the trade secrets for fixing faults in your physique. You've learned a selection of advanced technical tricks to modify exercises for maximum effect. You've also discovered ways to target muscles in hard-to-hit spots, and fine-tune your physique in areas of special needs such as symmetry and proportion. In the next chapter, you'll discover the doctor's prescription for muscle care, including tips for treating and preventing injury.

Sculpting Safely

Does the clang of iron plates get your adrenaline pumping? I bet you love a fierce challenge at the bench press or the squat rack. Am I right? First, two 45-pound (20.5 kg) plates on the bar, then four, then even more, gradually building up to your personal-best weight. Sweating under that barbell during the final few reps becomes a life-or-death situation, with only one winner. It's either you or the weight.

It's a great sense of achievement to beat that heavy barbell. And we all know that a powerful body is eye candy to casual onlookers. But there's one problem. All that heavy duty pushes your body to the limit. At the end of the day, there's always a bigger weight that's capable of demolishing your joints, tearing your tendons, or ripping your muscle in two.

No one is injury resistant, and no body is indestructible. Even Superman has a weakness. It doesn't matter how big or strong you are, there's always kryptonite lurking somewhere in the gym. So here's the thing: Never underestimate your potential for injury. The phrase "no pain, no gain" might be highlighted in the bodybuilder's bible, but it's not one of the 10 commandments of injury prevention.

Of all the potential pitfalls that prevent bodybuilding progress, injury throws the biggest wrench in the works and therefore deserves special attention. Most injuries can be prevented or treated if you take the right steps. One step not to take is to neglect or ignore the problem.

Like any other machine, your body demands care and attention. If you abuse the machine or neglect its upkeep, it won't function to the best of its ability. So let's talk about exercising safely. As the saying goes, an ounce of prevention is better than a pound of cure.

CAUSES OF INJURY

Several factors play roles in weight-training injury. The most common causes of injury include

- technical error,
- lifting too much weight,
- overtraining,
- poor equipment, and
- inexperience.

Technical error occurs when you're doing something wrong or performing an exercise with incorrect form (e.g., using inappropriate hand or foot spacing, arching your back, or swinging the weights). Forgetting to warm up before a workout also counts as a technical error. The technical tips that accompany the exercises in this book will help you maintain correct form.

Using a weight that's too heavy is a common mistake that leads to injury. Always choose a weight that allows you to perform at least six repetitions before failure. Make sure you have a spotter if you're under a barbell.

Too much exercise, or overtraining, is another common cause of injury. This situation arises when you train too long and your muscles become overfatigued, or when you exercise too often and don't give your body enough time to recover. The overfatigued or under-recovered muscle is a sitting duck for injury. To avoid overtraining, keep your workouts under an hour, and allow adequate rest in your workout schedule.

The type and location of weight-training equipment you choose also affect your chance of injury—in particular, whether you choose to train at home and whether you use free weights or machines. Surveys show that 40 percent of weight training injuries occur at home. Apparently, poor equipment and lack of supervision (no spotter) are to blame. When comparing machines and free weights, machines are safer. Two of three weight-training injuries involve free weights. This probably comes as no surprise. I bet most of you veteran lifters can recall getting trapped under a barbell bench press or dropping a heavy dumbbell on your foot. If your goal is to be safety conscious, I recommend that you join a good gym and strap yourself into their machines.

Injury rates are high among novices. It takes time and practice to master lifting techniques. However, inexperience does not plague just the newcomers to the gym. Whenever you try a new exercise, you become a temporary novice who needs to learn a new technique. You might have years of gym experience under your lifting belt, but if you've never done a deadlift, for instance, you've got to learn and practice the maneuver. If you don't respect the exercise during your first few sessions, you could end up with a nasty back injury. There's no substitute for the careful practice of new exercise techniques.

INJURY PREVENTION

If you've ever had an injury, you know that the forced period of inactivity is frustrating. Putting your workouts on hold while your injured body part heals can be a significant setback. Your fitness level and conditioning deteriorate, your strength diminishes, and your hard-earned muscle size melts away before your eyes. Not being able to exercise can make you irritable and depressed—workout withdrawal is real. You can avoid all this by taking precautions to reduce your chance of injury. Injury precautions should be a part of everyone's workout routine. Being safe makes perfect sense. Here are some tips to prevent injury:

- Warm up first with five minutes of cardio or a few minutes of cardio followed by a few minutes of stretching.
- Avoid massive weights. You must be able to perform at least six reps.
- Increase weight gradually, no more than 5 percent at a time.
- Keep workouts under an hour.
- Take one rest day each week.

- Cycle the intensity of your workouts (periodization).
- Train at a well-equipped gym.
- Use machines for greatest safety.
- Maintain correct technical form.
- Stop for sharp pain. Recognize the first signs of injury.

The risk of injury is greater at certain times. I call them windows for disaster. Such times are like driving on the freeway in heavy rain. Ease off the gas pedal. Exercise extreme caution when

- you're sick or more tired than usual,
- you train at a different time of day,
- you train during cold weather,
- you train at a new or unfamiliar gym, or
- you try a new exercise or a different piece of equipment.

Such times are probably not the greatest for trying for a new personal best. If you feel really tired or sick, substitute a scheduled weights workout with some gentle cardio or take an extra rest day. During cold weather, remember that your body needs a longer warm-up period and a few extra clothes to maintain body heat. Whenever you try a new exercise or equipment, there's a learning curve involved, so use lighter weights until you know what you're doing.

Torn Pec:
How can I avoid such an injury?

The pectoralis major muscle of the chest is made up of two anatomic sections, or heads. The upper clavicular head arises from the clavicle (collarbone), and the lower sternal head arises from the sternum (breastbone). The two heads pass outward across the chest wall and merge into a single tendon that attaches to the humerus bone in the upper arm. As the muscle inserts, the tendon twists so that the upper head attaches beneath the lower head. The tendon insertion is the site of most pec injuries. Why? Because this portion of the muscle is placed under excessive stretch as the weight is lowered during bench presses and chest flys. If you want to be safety conscious during these exercises, you need to pay close attention to five technical points: hand spacing, range of motion, rep speed, form, and resistance. So if you wish to avoid ripping your pec muscle, my suggestions are as follows:

- Use a shoulder-width grip during barbell bench presses (avoid wider grips).
- Do not lower the dumbbells too far during flys.
- Avoid fast negative reps.
- Do not bounce the weight off your chest.
- Use a weight that you can safely handle for at least six reps.

Injury First Aid

What should you do if you get injured? The first aid treatment for any injury aims to relieve pain, inflammation, and swelling. Follow six simple steps, which you can remember by the acronym PRICED (protect, rest, ice, compression, elevation, drugs):

- **Protect.** Stop the offending exercise immediately to prevent further damage from occurring.
- **Rest.** Restrict the use of the injured limb. When the injury involves your hip, knee, or ankle, walk only if absolutely necessary, and use a cane or crutches to minimize the weight placed on the leg.
- **Ice.** Apply an ice pack to the painful area for 10 to 15 minutes, repeating three or four times each day during the first 48 hours after injury.
- **Compression.** An elastic support keeps swelling to a minimum. Compression should not be too tight and must be removed intermittently to allow blood circulation. There's no need to wear the support when sleeping at night.
- **Elevation.** Elevating the limb uses gravity to improve blood flow back to the heart, aiding drainage of the fluid that causes swelling. The higher the elevation, the better the fluid drainage.
- **Drugs.** An anti-inflammatory medication, such as ibuprofen, helps relieve pain. Always read the label first, and follow the instructions. I usually recommend 400 mg of ibuprofen three times a day for a week after injury. Many anti-inflammatories are not recommended for people with stomach ulcers, asthma, or bleeding disorders.

You need to recognize the first signs of injury. Learn to distinguish the sharp pain arising from a joint or tendon from the burning ache of muscle fatigue. Any sharp pain is a warning sign saying back off or slow down. The safest response for sharp pain is to stop. Quit that exercise or even your whole workout. Follow the PRICED treatment procedure. Go home, apply some ice to the painful area, and take an anti-inflammatory medication. If the pain persists, see your doctor. Don't risk making the injury worse. Be attentive. Listen to the signals your body is sending. Treat any pain with respect.

If the pain, swelling, or bruising is severe, it's better to seek medical attention sooner rather than later. If you want an accurate diagnosis and the best treatment, there's no substitute for a proper medical evaluation. This involves a careful physical exam and an X-ray of the injured area to rule out a bone fracture. Further tests such as an ultrasound or MRI scan can help evaluate damage to the soft tissues of muscle, tendon, and ligament. The correct diagnosis is necessary for choosing the most effective treatment.

Tips for Trouble-Free Tendons

Tendons are cordlike connections that attach your muscles to bone. Without tendons, your muscles are useless chunks of meat. Tendon injury is a real concern for anyone who lifts heavy weights on a regular basis. Having said that, human tendons are remarkably strong—about half the strength of a stainless steel cable. The strength of a tendon depends on its size, and a 1 cm thick tendon can support a weight of more than 1,000 pounds (450 kg). Lifting weights improves tendon strength, but the adaptive change in tendon tissue occurs at a slower rate than the strength increase in the attached muscle.

When it comes to tendon protection, science indicates that the force transmitted through a tendon is affected by the *direction* of muscle contraction (positive or negative) and the *speed* at which the load is moved (fast or slow). A fast negative motion is potentially the most damaging to the tendon. Irrespective of the weight lifted, the stress through any tendon is larger during the negative phase of the movement, and even more so when the weight is lowered quickly. Even though a tendon is almost half as strong as a steel cable, this crucial structure is vulnerable to injury whenever you lift weights. In fact, the most common injury sustained in any gym is a tendon strain. Now if you do not want to be the owner of a painful damaged tendon that places your workouts on hold for weeks, there are some simple steps you can follow to ensure tendon health. You can reduce your chance of tendon injury with some simple strategic principles, as follows:

1. Warm up thoroughly before you work out. Increasing the blood flow and generating some warmth in the tissues is essential to prevent unwanted injury.

2. Avoid overstretching the muscle or tendon during exercise (e.g., lowering the weight too far during a chest fly). An extreme stretch under load can literally tear the tissue.

3. Perform slow, controlled repetitions. Fast reps, especially during the negative phase, place excessive stress on the muscle and tendon.

4. Avoid weights that are too heavy. The heavier the weight, the greater the risk of injury; it's much safer to keep your reps at six or more for each set.

5. Allow adequate rest between workouts. If you exercise the same muscle group several times per week, inadequate recovery time will result in overuse tendinitis.

6. Ensure an adequate daily intake of vitamin C (500 mg). This vitamin is critical for collagen—the substance that provides structural strength in muscle and tendon.

7. Try supplementing your diet with glucosamine (1,500 mg daily). This essential building block for cartilage can help reduce joint pains and arthritis.

8. Avoid smoking. Smoking restricts oxygen supply and expedites the aging process in numerous body tissues, tendons included.

MUSCLE CRAMPS

A cramp is a painful muscle spasm caused by a prolonged involuntary muscle contraction. It is sometimes caused by an imbalance of salts in the body, but it is more often a result of fatigue, imperfect posture, or stress. Cramps may also be linked to an underlying medical condition such as diabetes, poor circulation, thyroid disorders, and low calcium. Cases of persistent cramps sometimes require treatment with medication such as quinine. In athletes, cramps usually result from muscle fatigue or from dehydration during or after prolonged exercise. Although the *exact* cause is poorly understood, most cramps are self-limiting, and the painful spasm resolves once the exercise is discontinued. The most effective immediate treatment of a cramp is to release the knotted muscle by passive stretching. To keep this disabling problem from cramping your style, try the following suggestions.

1. Stretch: Static (nonballistic) stretching, before and after you work out, will prevent or alleviate muscle spasms.

2. Drink: Keep your body hydrated by drinking water regularly throughout the day and during your workout. An electrolyte drink or glass of fruit juice will help maintain sodium and potassium levels, and milk is an excellent source of calcium.

3. Decaffeinate: Since caffeine is a stimulant that can make cramps worse, you'd best stick to decaf if you drink coffee or tea.

4. Keep it short: Prevent excessive fatigue or dehydration by keeping your workout time under an hour.

5. Rest: Muscles need rest to repair the damage inflicted by an intense workout, and your body will perform better when you get adequate sleep.

6. Take a hot bath: Heat relaxes muscles and eases postworkout spasms. So go ahead and soak yourself!

STRETCHING SAFELY

A full range of motion is usually synonymous with good technical form when it comes to weight training. However, your body's anatomy *is* pushed to the limit at the extremes of joint motion, and it is well known that muscles are most vulnerable at full stretch—especially with added resistance. In my opinion, a "safer not to overstretch" policy is wise when lifting heavy during certain exercises. For example, a full stretch during chest flys dramatically increases unwanted stress across the shoulder joint and risks tearing the pectoralis muscle. A similar situation arises during preacher curls when the biceps tendon is fully stretched at the end of the downward phase. In both these circumstances, it is the tensile strength of the tendon that supports the weight, not the contractile strength of the muscle. Biomechanically, a shorter range of motion is definitely safer than a full stretch. This principle is particularly important for older lifters because muscles tend to become stiffer and less elastic with age. If you want to be safer when going for a full stretch, use a lighter weight.

JOINT PROTECTION

There are two things that can aggravate *healthy* joints: injury and obesity. Injury can damage the smooth surface of the joints, and being overweight can wear down the cartilage lining. Over time, both circumstances can result in arthritis, with accompanying joint pain and stiffness. These are well-established medical facts. Now let's apply this information to your time lifting at the gym. First of all, you are more likely to sustain an injury using heavy weights. Second of all, heavy weights increase the chance of grinding down the cartilage cushion inside your joints. So when it comes to aggravating your joints, heavy lifting carries the greatest risk. It follows then that a gentle jog on the treadmill is much less traumatic to your joints than grinding out a few reps with 500 pounds (225 kg) on the squat bar. Now I'm not suggesting we all become treadmill trotters. But we should strive to train safely—*pump muscles, don't grind joints.*

A question I'm often asked is whether weight training increases your risk of developing arthritis. Well, *osteoarthritis* is an affliction characterized by joint pain and stiffness that gets worse with age. The cartilage lining the joints has worn down, and the diagnosis is usually confirmed by way of an X-ray. In causative terms, osteoarthritis may be inherited, be inflicted by injury, or result from overuse. Despite being much safer than most injury-prone sports, lifting heavy weights can cause joint injury and over time may wear down the cartilage lining of your joints. The degree of wear and subsequent risk of arthritis are dependent on the amount of weight and the length of time spent performing the activity. Unfortunately, there are no specific safety guidelines and no exact time frame. But if you lift several hundred pounds every week for 10 years or more, chances are your joints will wear down. This consequence is similar to tire wear on any vehicle. The more you drive the quicker the tires deteriorate, and the tires wear down more if the vehicle carries a heavy load. Best advice for those who like to lift? If you want to avoid painful joints, use the following guidelines:

1. Select a weight that allows you to perform at least six reps.
2. Feel a pump in the muscle, not pain in the joint.
3. Cycle the intensity, and alternate heavy days with lighter workouts.
4. Allow adequate time between heavy days to give your joints some rest.
5. Avoid high-risk movements such as deep squats, behind-the-neck presses, and so on.
6. Employ variety in your workouts, switching between barbell, dumbbells, cables, and machines.
7. Downsize your workouts as you get older, and don't lift as much weight.
8. Try supplementing your diet with glucosamine.

NECK SAFETY

Muscle spasms in the neck area are common. Why? Because these muscles are under constant tension—the neck muscles work constantly to hold the head up, and the trapezius works to support your upper limbs. If you lift weights regularly, those overdeveloped traps are prone to spasms and cramps. Typically, the affected muscles are tender to the touch, and you'll often feel a lump, or knot, in the muscle. Other causes of neck pain include a trapped nerve or neck arthritis. Here are some suggestions to avoid or alleviate a nagging neck ache.

1. Keep your head straight, and avoid arching or turning your neck during all exercises.
2. Use padding when you support a barbell across your traps (e.g., during squats).
3. Cut back on exercises that target the traps directly (e.g., shrugs, deadlifts).
4. Make sure you sleep with proper neck support and a correctly sized pillow, and avoid cold air drafts such as an open window or fan.
5. Be aware of your posture when driving and during working hours.
6. Gently stretch the neck muscles before and after each workout. Turn your head toward your right shoulder to feel a stretch in the left trapezius; look toward the left shoulder to stretch the right trapezius; and place your chin on your chest to stretch the middle portion of the muscle. Hold each stretch for 10 seconds; rest and repeat until your neck muscles feel loose and supple. Rotating the head in a circular motion is another way to help loosen up the neck muscles.

SHOULDER SAFETY

The key to building strong shoulders that survive the test of time without injury is knowing your anatomy. So let's review some anatomical facts and devise sensible suggestions for shoulder safety and longevity.

Fact 1: The shoulder is the most mobile joint in your body. But with this mechanical freedom comes vulnerability. Your shoulder joint is not designed to lift weights behind the plane of your body.

Suggestion: Avoid behind-the-neck presses and pull-downs, and keep your hands in front where you can see them.

Fact 2: The shoulder has a delicate inner sleeve of muscles called the rotator cuff. Because this inner layer is barely visible, it is often neglected at the gym. This is a big mistake because a weak rotator cuff is easily injured, causing pain and disability.

Suggestion: Begin every shoulder workout with rotator cuff exercises as part of your warm-up.

Fact 3: The deltoid muscle has three sections: front (anterior), side (lateral), and rear (posterior). It is very important to develop the deltoid in proportion because muscle imbalance can result in injury. Routines that rely heavily on pressing movements favor overdevelopment of the front deltoid.

Suggestion: Pay equal attention to all three heads of the deltoid muscle, making sure to include side and rear lateral raise exercises.

Shoulder pain is an occupational hazard for anyone who works out. The reason? Rotator cuff tendinitis, or *impingement*—a condition that causes pain when you raise your arm overhead. As you raise your arm up and out, the space between the shoulder bones gets smaller. And if your rotator cuff tendon gets squashed

Clicking Concern: Why does my shoulder click when I do shoulder exercises?

A clicking joint is not a cause for concern *unless* you feel pain or experience disability. At the shoulder, *painless* clicking is usually caused by the rotator cuff tendons moving back and forth over the bone. Typically, this phenomenon does not cause injury. You can minimize shoulder noise by warming up adequately and by keeping your rotator cuff strong (using the exercises described in chapter 14, pages 178–180). However, if symptoms persist or your joint becomes painful, loose, or stiff, I'd recommend that you see a medical doctor. You may require an X-ray or MRI scan to rule out problematic causes of a clicking shoulder such as a torn labrum, an unstable joint, or arthritis.

against the bone, the tendon will become inflamed and painful. It's as if you were squeezing the tendon in the jaws of a wrench with every rep! Bodybuilders tend to neglect the relatively small rotator cuff muscles because they are barely visible. The resulting muscle imbalance leaves the weakened rotator cuff vulnerable to injury. During your shoulder workout at the gym, pain-provoking exercises typically include behind-the-neck presses and upright rows. Lateral raises may cause pain if your hands pass above shoulder level. Whenever you feel pain, it means you are irritating the inflamed rotator cuff tendon. And the tendon won't heal until you stop tweaking it.

Rules for Rotator Cuff Survival

So how can you avoid provoking your shoulder pain at the gym? Pick exercises that do not place your arm into a position of impingement. To guide you, I have created a set of rules for rotator cuff survival:

Rule 1: Strengthen the rotator cuff muscles.

Rule 2: Always keep your hands in full view to the front.

Rule 3: Do not raise your elbows above shoulder level.

Rule 4: Do not use a wide grip when you press.

Rule 5: Avoid exercises that provoke pain (e.g., behind-the-neck movements).

I'd also recommend some *modifications* to your exercise choices to avoid those exercises that provoke your pain. Check out the following list of exercises that are typically painful for someone with rotator cuff tendinitis. Try substituting the painful exercises in table 16.1 with a corresponding exercise that is less likely to inflict pain.

Table 16.1 Exercise Guide for a Painful Shoulder

Painful exercise	Painless exercise
Behind-the-neck shoulder press	Front shoulder press
Upright row	Side lateral raise
Behind the neck pull-down	Front pull-down
Incline bench press	Decline bench press
Free weights	Machine exercises

To avoid rotator cuff impingement, suitable exercises to incorporate into your shoulder workouts include lateral deltoid raises, rear deltoid flys, front deltoid raises, and front shoulder presses.

Correct Cuff Exercises

When it comes to strengthening the rotator cuff, many trainers demonstrate the exercises with the elbow elevated at 90 degrees, perpendicular to the body, in the high-five position. However, in my opinion as a shoulder surgeon, this is not the ideal position to work the rotator cuff muscle for two scientific reasons. First, when the rotator cuff muscles contract, the humerus bone of the upper arm is rotated outward (by infraspinatus and teres minor) or inward (by subscapularis). With the elbow close to the side of your body, the mechanical axis of these muscles is anatomic. In other words, this is their preferred biomechanical plane. Performing the rotation exercises with the elbow elevated at 90 degrees is a less favorable position for these muscles.

Second, if you have a shoulder injury, the high-five position makes the joint vulnerable. Performing exercises with the arm in this position can irritate the rotator cuff, causing impingement, or tendinitis. So, performing rotator cuff exercises in the high-five position can in fact *create* a shoulder problem. What's more, if you are trying to rehabilitate a damaged rotator cuff, performing the exercises with the elbow elevated is counterproductive and can make the injury worse. Bottom line: If you wish to build your rotator cuff in the safest biomechanical way, you'll choose my method. Perform the internal and external rotation exercises with your elbow close to the side of your body (as described in chapter 14) using a cable pulley or a rubber exercise band.

ELBOW SAFETY

At the gym, elbow pain is typically due to tendinitis—specifically, inflammation of the forearm extensor or flexor muscles. *Lateral epicondylitis*, or tennis elbow, usually results from an overuse injury to the extensor muscles of the forearm and causes pain in the outer elbow. *Medial epicondylitis*, or golfer's elbow, is an overuse injury to the flexor muscles of the forearm and causes pain over the inner elbow. Any activity that requires a strong grip can provoke elbow tendinitis. So if you are frequently gripping a heavy dumbbell or barbell at the gym, your elbow may be at risk. Treatment for elbow tendinitis typically involves a short period of rest, avoiding activities that provoke the pain. You don't have to quit upper body workouts. I recommend *modifying* your training program to allow the injury time to heal. Here are my suggestions:

- Avoid exercises that provoke pain.
- Utilize a thumbless grip.
- Choose machines where the force is transmitted through elbow pads.
- Use wrist straps during back exercises.
- Strengthen the damaged tendon with wrist curls using a lightweight dumbbell.

SPINE SAFETY

Probably the most common hazard in any gym is back injury. Why? Because weightlifting places enormous stress on the spine. When you think about it, the lower back is used in almost *every* workout, even when you're just loading weights onto a barbell or grabbing dumbbells off the rack. During any workout, you can injure your back by one of several mechanisms. The first is a compressive force when the spine supports a weight (e.g., during squats or overhead presses). The second is when the spine bends forward (e.g., during deadlifts or bent-over rows). The third is when the spine is subjected to an uneven one-sided load (e.g., during lunges or overhead dumbbell presses).

Typically, back injury occurs during a standing exercise when the spine is unsupported. In most cases injury results from a simple mistake such as insufficient warm-up, lifting too much weight, overfatigue, or technical error. When your back supports a loaded squat bar, the discs between the bones of your spinal column flatten and bulge out—just like when you squeeze a tennis ball between the palms of your hands. Repeated heavy loads over time can cause the soft-cushion discs to bulge permanently. And when this happens, the disc pushes on the nerves passing through the spine, causing pain in the buttocks and leg—a condition known as *sciatica*. If you keep provoking the problem, the disc may burst, and you could require surgery. However, if you stop loading your spine with heavy weights, the disc bulge can subside.

The most common lower back injury is a sprain of the lumbar ligaments. The pain is felt off-center to the right or left of the lower spine and is made worse by bending forward (spine flexion). Pain from a slipped disc travels into the buttock and down the back of the leg. With an injured back, safety should be your main concern, not slam-dunking big weights. It is safer to avoid any exercise that transmits a load across your spine. A good rule of thumb is to select seated or lying exercises using machines. Choose your exercises wisely, and whenever possible perform the movement seated while supporting your spine with a backrest. A good exercise for lower back strength is lumbar extensions. When you perform this exercise, avoid arching your spine. Raise your torso until it's parallel with the floor, but do not hyperextend. Here are my top 10 tips for avoiding back injury.

1. Always warm up before you work out.
2. Strengthen your lower back using lumbar extensions.
3. Remember to keep your abdominal muscles strong.
4. Wear a supportive belt when needed.
5. Pay close attention to correct exercise technique.
6. Keep your spine straight, and avoid arching.
7. Avoid *excessive* axial loads on the spine (e.g., during squats and overhead presses).
8. Use caution during bent-over exercises (e.g., deadlifts and bent-over rows).
9. Make good use of machines, since they tend to be safer than free weights.
10. Perform seated exercises, and use backrests or chest pads as often as possible.

Some safer spine-friendly exercise suggestions for those with low backache are listed in table 16.2.

Table 16.2   Spine-Friendly Exercises to Avoid Backache

What's OUT	What's IN
Squat	Leg press, leg extension
Deadlift	Lumbar extension
Bent-over row	Seated machine row
Overhead press	Seated press with a back support

HIP SAFETY

At the gym, hip pain may be due to a mild case of hip joint arthritis or a groin strain—an injury to the adductor muscle of the inner thigh. While the injury heals, you will need to make intelligent exercise choices to create a workout that maintains leg muscle strength without provoking the pain. The key is to avoid weight transmission directly across the hip. Activities that stress the hip joint include running, squats, lunges, and deadlifts. Lower limb exercises that spare the hip region include leg extensions, leg curls, seated calf raises, and cycling on a stationary bike. Lightweight leg presses may also be possible provided the movement does not induce pain. You can also try the following suggestions to *avoid* hip or groin injury.

1. Stretch before and during your leg workout.
2. Warm up using a stationary bike.
3. Avoid a wide stance during squats and leg presses.
4. Point your toes and knees straight ahead.
5. Take shorter steps when performing lunges.
6. Strengthen hip muscles using the leg adductor–abductor machine.

KNEE SAFETY

A *noisy* knee is a very common symptom if you exercise regularly. Many people experience a grinding or clicking sensation as their knees bend—while climbing stairs or arising from a squat position. The symptom usually indicates a softening or thinning of the cartilage behind the kneecap, known as *chondromalacia patella*. This condition tends to occur with increasing age as the knee cartilage wears down. But it can also arise when there is a family predisposition or after an injury to the kneecap during sports. Provided that you're not experiencing any pain, the clicking noise does not require any specific treatment.

A *painful* knee in athletic people may be due to kneecap injury, patellar tendinitis, or a torn meniscus (the cartilage cushion between the bones of the knee joint). The meniscus can be damaged by a sudden twist of the knee or a deep squat. When torn, it typically causes symptoms of pain, swelling, clicking, and locking. At the gym, expect your knee pain to be provoked by squatting, leg presses, and lunges, especially if the knee bends more than 90 degrees. A painful knee will of course make leg workouts somewhat tricky. You can try training legs, but utilize short-arc movements so as not to bend your knee beyond 90 degrees. Wherever possible, perform a seated exercise rather than a standing one. Assess each exercise on a trial basis, and if the movement hurts, don't do it. You probably won't have difficulty with leg extensions, leg curls, or a stationary bike. But you should use caution when performing deep knee bends during squats, leg presses, and lunges. Here are some suggestions to minimize knee symptoms during leg workouts.

1. Warm up your knees first by spending 5 to 10 minutes on the stationary bike.
2. Perform an isolation exercise, such as leg extensions, at the beginning of your leg workout.
3. Avoid bending the knee beyond 90 degrees during squats or leg presses, restricting the range of knee motion to a short arc.
4. Do not use elastic knee wraps, since such devices compress the kneecap against the femur bone, making the problem worse.

Shin Splints: I like to run, but I get shin splints. Is there anything I can do to prevent them?

The term *shin splints* refers to symptoms of exercise-induced leg pain. This condition is usually brought on by repetitive activities during high-impact aerobic exercises, such as jogging or running. The obvious solution to this problem is to avoid the repetitive stress that is provoking it, and the leg pain will go away. Now that doesn't mean you cannot get a good cardio workout. My recommendation would be *nonimpact* aerobic activities. Good alternatives to running include the stationary bike, elliptical trainer, and stair climber as well as swimming. Walking on a treadmill is a low-impact activity that might also be suitable. Most cases of shin splints will heal after a month or two of rest, restricted weight bearing, and modified activities.

Even though weight training is one of the safest forms of exercise, you can still hurt yourself at the gym. Incorporate my tips for exercising *safely* and you will reduce your chance of injury when you work out. In the next chapter, we discuss other pitfalls that can impede your body-sculpting progress, and you'll learn simple survival strategies for maintaining your perfect physique.

Survival Strategies for the Peak Physique

I t's easier to maintain the changes you make to your body than it is to create them in the first place. Bodybuilding is like hiking on a mountain. With each difficult step upward you make progress, but once you've got your footing, it doesn't take much effort to hold your ground.

There are many paths up the mountain. Depending on your goals, you can head in the direction of muscle mass or switch your destination toward fat loss. Providing you stay on the well-trodden paths, you'll avoid sliding back down the slippery slope. Still, you're bound to encounter a few unforeseen obstacles along the route. There will be demons—overtraining, injury, lack of discipline, loss of motivation—perched on your shoulder, tempting you toward disaster. What you need to ward off these demons is a maintenance plan, a strategy to thwart disaster and guide you around the obstacles. Maintaining your body is easy if you know how.

A perfect physique requires several key ingredients mixed in the right measures, brewed in the best environment, and nurtured over time. None of these steps can be left to chance. If you neglect even the smallest detail, you won't turn out a classic sculpture. Use the following 12-point problem–solution checklist to prevent pitfalls and remedy the problems that impede your bodybuilding progress.

INCORPORATE VARIETY

The problem: muscle boredom.

The solution: muscle confusion.

We've all heard that variety is the spice of life. Well, this pearl of wisdom applies to your muscles, too. You see, muscles are incredibly adaptive to exercise, and they respond to one type of training for only a limited time. Persisting with the same routine indefinitely condemns you to physique stagnation. Your muscles get bored. Sticking to the same exercises out of habit or an unwillingness to change keeps you fixed at the same level of development.

A solution to muscle boredom is muscle confusion. To break free of a training plateau, shock your muscles by asking them to do something they haven't done before. Changing your exercise stimulus forces your muscles to adapt to new demands.

Incorporating variety into your exercise program keeps your workout fresh. Change your exercises or the structure of your workout. Confuse your muscles by giving them a challenge they haven't faced before. Avoid the same old routine; keep your muscles guessing.

With each workout, make small changes to the exercise content and order. For example, you can do bench presses using a standard barbell, a pair of dumbbells, or a machine. You can do biceps curls using a straight bar, dumbbells, cables, or a machine. Changing the way you do an exercise from one workout to the next forces your muscles to adapt on a regular basis. Your muscles don't become stale and you won't get bored from doing the same old exercises.

Keep a pool of your favorite exercises for each muscle group, and select a different movement each time you work out. The best workouts are the ones that keep challenging your muscles.

SCULPT PROPORTIONALLY

The problem: a lagging body part.

The solution: priority training.

An eye-catching physique requires more than just mass. Individual muscle groups must be developed in proportion. Sure, every bodybuilder wants big biceps—those huge arms are always on display in the "shop window." But if your bulging biceps overshadow your chest and shoulder development, you're not displaying a crafted physique. Heads may turn at the sight of bulging muscles, but jaws drop in the presence of sculpted body work.

Muscle Memory: Is there such a thing as muscle memory?

If you've worked out before, getting *back* in shape is definitely easier than starting from scratch. We tend to call this phenomenon *muscle memory*. Basically it's the result of previous skill, experience, and knowledge. If you've learned a *skill* before, your body memorizes the basic technical capability to perform that activity, despite a layoff. Plus with previous *experience*, you *know* how to get your body in shape. It's like riding a bicycle—if you've done it before, it's easy to get rolling again. The time it takes to get back in shape depends on your age and current physical condition. Despite the advantage of muscle memory, the older you are and more out of shape you are, the longer it will take.

A balanced, proportioned physique looks amazing, but it makes biomechanical sense, too. Muscle imbalances are a fast track to injury. A neglected rotator cuff is a prime example. Ignore these muscles, and a pair of painful shoulders will soon be yours. Instead of blasting away with set after intense set of arm builders, train all your body parts with equal attention.

Despite your diligence to train each muscle group with equal intensity, you might discover that some body parts respond better to exercise than others. Even professional bodybuilders suffer the plague of lagging body parts. Sometimes the culprit is subconscious neglect, but more often the problem is genetic. Certain muscle groups are just wired differently. Some people are blessed with big arms; others are born with king-sized calves. It's worth being objective and recognizing the chink in your armor—you can fix the lagging muscle group through priority training.

Prioritizing the weak area of your physique means paying the area special attention and focus. There are three ways to do this. First, train the underdeveloped body part at the beginning of your workout when your energy level is highest. Second, relocate the weak muscle group to the beginning of a workout week when your body is fresh from the rest period over the weekend. Third, simply work the lagging muscle more than you work the others.

CYCLE YOUR WORKOUTS

The problem: overtraining.

The solution: periodization.

To benefit from regular exercise, you need to do 30 minutes of physical activity at least three times a week. That's bare minimum. On the flip side, if you're exercising for more than an hour each day, seven days a week, you're doing too much. It's virtually impossible for your body to recover fully from each workout on this kind of a schedule, so you won't gain muscle size or strength. Doing too much exercise is counterproductive; it leads to a state of overtraining. When this happens, you stop making progress, get weaker, and leave yourself wide open to injury. Remember that your muscles must recover from the exercise stimulus in order to reap the benefits. More is not necessarily better. And don't make your regimen more complicated than it needs to be. Keep it simple. If you think you're overtraining, take this little quiz in table 17.1 to be sure.

Table 17.1 Are You Overtraining?

1. Do you always feel tired?	Yes	No
2. Are you losing muscle size?	Yes	No
3. Have you lost strength?	Yes	No
4. Are your muscles tender?	Yes	No
5. Has your appetite decreased?	Yes	No
6. Do you have difficulty sleeping?	Yes	No
7. Do your workouts lack energy?	Yes	No
8. Do you lack motivation?	Yes	No

If you answered yes to more than three questions, you might be overtraining. If you answered yes to more than five questions, you're very likely overtraining.

The solution to overtraining is periodization. Periodization is the process of cycling the intensity and format of your workouts. This technique gives you flexibility to make adjustments in your training regimen. You can make cyclic changes over short monthly intervals or on a longer seasonal basis.

In the short term, you should cycle your workout intensity. After four to six weeks of high-intensity training, ease off the gas pedal and reduce intensity for a couple of weeks. This periodic downtime provides two major benefits. First, your

Weather Effect: Does the weather affect my workout?

The environmental temperature does affect your training. As any seasoned bodybuilder will tell you, working out in a warm gym means your body needs less time to warm up, and your muscles are less likely to get cold between sets. By minimizing warm-up time and maintaining body heat, warmer temperatures benefit short, intense bodybuilding-style workouts. Heat will also boost your heart rate and make you breathe heavier than you would in a cooler environment. The upside of this extra exertion is that you'll burn more calories in less time. The downside is that hot weather can also wear you out quicker, cutting your workout short or reducing workout intensity. On the flip side, in a cold gym your body needs more time to warm up, and your muscles can cool down quickly between sets. A cold environment carries an increased risk of injury, especially when lifting heavy weights. However, a cooler temperature may allow you to work out at a higher intensity for a longer duration, resulting in a greater overall calorie burn. The bottom line in this debate is probably that warmer is better for building muscle, whereas cooler is better for cardio.

body gets a rest, which helps prevent overtraining and injury. Second, your mind gets a rest, which helps maintain motivation. Intense workouts are extremely demanding; downtime helps prevent burnout.

In the long term, you can change the focus of your training program on a seasonal basis. For instance, you might choose to bulk up during the winter season using the mass generator program (chapter 7). In the spring, you could switch to the body fat blitz program (chapter 10). During the summer, you can flip over to the hybrid hard body program (chapter 14) to look your best on the beach. Then during the fall, select a period of low intensity to give your body some respite.

It doesn't matter how you cycle the intensity of your workouts or when you switch from one program to another. The important thing is that you do incorporate periodization in your game plan. Changing the intensity and focus of your workouts on a regular basis is a key factor for continued progress as well as for preventing overtraining.

STAY NUTRITIONALLY SOUND

The problem: using the wrong fuel.

The solution: dietary discipline.

Anything you put in your mouth should serve a nutritional purpose, not just satisfy your hunger or appeal to your taste buds. Don't waste your calorie count on useless junk. For instance, a doughnut has no real nutritional benefit. Sure, it tastes good and provides a small sugar rush, but that glazed ring of candy becomes a spare tire around your waist. It has no muscle-building benefit at all. You wouldn't pour sugar into your car's gas tank, would you? If you're going to eat something, make it worthwhile. Junk food is body pollution. You don't litter anywhere else, so why put litter in your body?

To prevent nutrition setbacks, use dietary discipline. If you're not gaining muscle or losing fat, the first thing to do is review your calorie intake and check your daily calorie requirement. Then check the content of your diet and the ratio of protein, carbohydrate, and fat. Make sure you comply with the recommendations in your diet plan. There's no quick-fix diet or magic pill for fat loss and muscle gain. If you want healthy, lasting results, you need to change your lifestyle. Follow these tips to keep your diet on track:

Keep a cookbook Writing down your personal diet plan is essential for success. Calculate your daily calorie requirement (body weight in pounds × 10, or body weight in kilograms × 22), and consume six small meals at three- to four-hour intervals during the day. Write down your meal schedule, record the content of each meal, and stick to the plan. To facilitate fat loss, the ratio of macronutrients in your diet should be about 50 percent protein, 40 percent carbohydrate, and 10 percent fat. Consume at least 1 gram of protein per pound (.5 kg) of body weight each day.

Eat clean to be lean Clean food is devoid of any unnecessary additives and thus has no hidden calories. For example, a plain grilled chicken breast is clean, whereas a piece of fried chicken in breadcrumbs is not. Similarly, a baked potato is clean, but a plate of fries is loaded with fat calories. Keeping your diet simple makes it easier to monitor calories. Processed foods such as mayonnaise contain lots of salt, fat, and preservatives. Sauces and flavorings should be low fat and used sparingly.

Keep it simple The focus of your attention should be on the protein, carbohydrate, fat, and calorie content of food. Don't get bogged down by small, unnecessary details. It wastes your time and distracts you from the big picture.

Shop to succeed Don't go to the grocery store hungry. Make a list and stick to it. If it's not on your list of authorized foods, don't even pick it up. When your house is free of junk food, you'll be less likely to have a damaging snack attack. Keep junk food out of sight, out of mind.

Read the label Calculating food portions and calories is easy if you read the product label. Pay close attention to what constitutes a serving because the calorie content is based on this amount. If a product doesn't have a label with nutrition facts, don't eat it unless it came from a tree or the ground.

Pack a snack Eating small meals every three to four hours means you'll sometimes eat outside your home. Go prepared! Pack several small meals or snacks to take to work. Meal-replacement drinks, protein shakes or bars, and fruit are useful for this purpose. Pack enough supplies to avoid hunger pangs and the temptation of junk food.

Consume everything in moderation No matter what you eat, never gorge yourself until your belly pops your buttons off. One helping is enough. Stuffing yourself bloats your belly and protrudes your waistline. Excess calories consumed at one sitting get stored as fat.

Think before you drink Your average eight-ounce (240 ml) beverage contains at least 100 calories, whether it's soda, fruit juice, milk, or beer. During the course of the day, it's easy to drink away almost half of your daily calorie intake.

The solution to this pollution is water. Remember that 70 percent of your muscle is water, and you should drink at least a gallon (4 L) of water every day to maintain hydration. The caffeine in coffee and tea can aid fat loss, and these beverages are low in calories if you don't add milk or sugar. If you crave soda, make sure your choice is low in calories.

Be prepared when dining out   Eating healthfully at a restaurant is not impossible. Substitute unhealthful side dishes such as fries with a small salad or steamed rice. Ask for sauces and dressings to be placed on the side. Dip your fork into the dressing and then take a bite of your food. It's a great way to keep the flavor without getting the excess calories. If there are no substitutions, try to build a meal from the healthier single side orders on the menu. When all else fails, find another place to eat. Remember that you do have one cheat day per week. If you want to make dining out a feast to remember, use your cheat day to order whatever you want.

Use supplements intelligently   Eating a nutritious diet is far more important than the supplements you take. Supplements add to your diet; they don't take the place of it. For instance, meal-replacement drinks are convenient when you're on the go. Protein shakes top off your protein intake, and liquid is easily digested when you replenish after a workout. A bite or two from a low-carbohydrate protein bar is an acceptable way to curb cravings between meals. A multivitamin or mineral supplement helps prevent dietary deficiencies. Adequate consumption of vitamins B, C, and E aids exercise and recovery.

Set short-term goals   Instead of thinking of your nutrition plan as a diet, think of it as changing the way you eat. Take your time and be patient. Start by setting daily goals. Eliminate desserts, candy, and other unhealthful snacks. Replace soda with water. Select low-fat alternatives. Then tackle the goals that might take longer to accomplish. Gradually cut back on carbohydrate and increase protein in your diet. Monitor your progress with a weekly weight check on the bathroom scale and a monthly body fat measurement with a skinfold caliper. Take small steps in the right direction.

Don't get caught in a fad   Forget about secrets or shortcuts in dieting. There aren't any. Most fad diets work only in the short term. If you want to lose weight and keep it off, you have to make lasting lifestyle changes. Learn to cook, shop, and dine in a healthful way, and those pounds will stay off.

Forgive your mistakes   We all have our vices. If you fall off the wagon and engage in a weekend of beer and pizza, don't panic. If you make a mistake, you can't really compensate by overexercising or starving yourself. Let mistakes be bygones, get back on schedule, and keep moving forward. Don't let setbacks or mistakes slow you down, but do try to learn from your indiscretions.

GET YOUR SLEEP

The problem: lethargy.

The solution: rest and recovery.

If you feel constantly tired or lack energy for your workouts, check your sleeping habits. Today's dollar-driven, fast-paced lifestyle leaves many of us in a state of chronic sleep deprivation. People don't sleep enough to recharge their batteries, which results in lethargy and suboptimal levels of performance. Remember that growth and recovery happen while you sleep.

If you're exercising regularly, your body needs seven to eight hours of sleep each night to allow repair mechanisms to do their job. Adequate sleep is especially important if you're trying to build muscle. If you have to rise at the crack of dawn to get to work, make sure you go to bed early the night before. Resist the temptation to stay up late socializing or watching TV. Make getting enough sleep a high priority. If you can't fit in eight hours of sleep overnight, seize any opportunity during the day to take a 30- to 60-minute power nap to recharge your batteries. You'll feel more refreshed for the rest of the day. Whatever happens, don't let chronic sleep deprivation hamper your progress.

INCREASE INTENSITY

The problem: lacking mass.

The solution: intensify.

If you're not packing on pounds of muscle, you're not putting enough effort into your training. When at the gym, do you train your butt off or just go through the motions? To make progress, you have to keep challenging yourself, continually pushing your body to new limits.

Muscle growth requires a hypertrophic stimulus. That means six to eight reps performed to failure. To continually challenge your muscles, train beyond failure with the techniques that generate added intensity (see chapter 11). Without intensity, muscles won't grow.

KEEP YOUR FOCUS

The problem: you're easily distracted.

The solution: stay focused.

If you want to benefit from your workouts, you simply can't waste time at the gym. To achieve the best results, keep your workouts short, sweet, and intense. When you're not lifting a weight, you're catching your breath and lining up the next exercise. There's no time for gossip or reading a book. If you waste more than two minutes between sets or exercises, you won't get your workout done on time. Before you know it, you're spending over an hour in the gym. No way can you fulfill your best workouts if you're constantly catching up on gossip. Oversocializing wastes precious gym time and extends your workouts needlessly.

If you're easily distracted, take steps to prevent it. Avoid making eye contact. Wear stereo headphones while you train to discourage interruptions. Get serious. Switch off your cell phone; there's nothing that can't wait 30 minutes while you complete your workout. An effective workout demands your full attention, so don't corrupt it.

STAY CLEAN

The problem: contamination.

The solution: just say no.

It goes without saying that alcohol and substance abuse affects your health and fitness. We're talking about recreational drugs here, not those prescribed for medical reasons by your doctor. Alcohol affects exercise performance and recovery. It's also a source of useless and unnecessary calories. It doesn't matter how meticulous you are with food intake; if you're drinking a few servings of alcohol every day, you won't reduce body fat. A few bottles of beer or some wine over the weekend won't hurt, but be moderate.

Cigarette smoking impairs lung function and reduces the oxygen supply to your muscles. You can't perform to the best of your abilities if you're polluting your lungs on a daily basis. Similarly, recreational drugs such as marijuana adversely affect exercise performance and your body's ability to recover. You can't become a high-performance machine if you're voluntarily contaminating your body.

For a whole host of health reasons, abstinence is best. If you want to make the best possible progress with your fitness goals, just say no to drugs and alcohol.

TAKE A SHORT BREAK

The problem: a lack of time.

The solution: downtime.

Your training commitment amounts to less than five hours per week. Even the busiest of work schedules can accommodate a daily 30-minute workout. However, there will be circumstances that interfere with gym time, including vacations, ill health, domestic obligations, work deadlines, and business trips. With careful planning, your muscle-building progress should not suffer.

Everyone needs downtime once in a while, and a short break from your workout schedule won't interfere with your progress. However, apply two rules when taking time-outs. First, they should last no longer than a week or two. Second, don't take them too frequently. Exercise and diet must be maintained on a regular basis. Your workout program is only as effective as your last bout of exercise, and your diet is only as healthy as your last meal. Muscles adapt to the demands placed on them. If you stop exercising, muscle shrinks and loses its strength.

A short interruption won't have adverse effects on your overall progress. If you stop exercising for a week, you won't lose significant muscle size or strength. In fact, a seven-day period of complete rest allows your body to restock muscle fuel and heal nagging injuries. Aches and pains disappear or diminish, and when you resume exercising, you'll feel stronger and more energetic. But there's a fine line between a short therapeutic rest and an extended layoff. Two weeks is probably the longest time you can safely take off without compromising strength and fitness. If you take a longer time-out, you'll lose conditioning, which makes it tough to get back on course when you resume your workouts.

If you stop exercising for longer than two weeks, your muscles atrophy and decrease in size and strength. Muscles don't turn to fat—this is physically impossible because muscle and fat are two completely different tissues. What happens when you stop exercising is that you continue eating the same amount of food, but you don't burn as many calories. The excess calories get stored as fat. If you want to avoid gaining weight when you stop exercising, reduce the amount of calories you consume to match your reduced calorie expenditure.

The bottom line is that a short time-out is acceptable when taken infrequently. You can allow yourself a week off every three to four months or a total of four weeks

Winter Colds: Should I be working out when I'm under the weather?

Runny nose, mild cough, and headache. Should we exercise when suffering from the common cold? Good question! Scientific study indicates that *moderate* exercise boosts the immune system, protecting against ill health and alleviating cold symptoms. On the other hand, *intense* bouts of exercise can depress immunity and have a detrimental effect. So it seems that working out while under the weather is safe, provided you don't overdo it. A word of caution, though: If you're suffering from a *severe* bout of influenza (fever, muscle pains, sore throat, and so on), you'd best avoid exercise and instead rest until symptoms pass. Here are some general guidelines for those with mild cold symptoms who wish to work out.

1. Reduce workout intensity using lighter weights.
2. Do not exercise to the point of exhaustion.
3. Cut back on workout volume by performing fewer sets and exercises.
4. Limit workout duration to about 30 minutes.
5. Substitute a weights session with some gentle cardio.
6. Do not train more than three times a week.
7. Drink plenty of fluids.
8. Supplement your diet with vitamin C.
9. Get adequate rest.
10. Take a symptomatic cold medication.

a year. If you let your exercise program or diet lapse for longer periods, you'll lose your conditioning. So, when you must call a time-out, use it wisely.

Another solution to a lack of time is a busybody workout. During times when family or work commitments become demanding, downsize your workout schedule to accommodate them. Staying in shape doesn't require as much time as most people think. Four 30-minute workouts each week are all you need to maintain an exercise commitment.

When your time is required elsewhere, you can make do with two simple 30-minute in-and-out workout routines. The first workout is indoor weight training aimed at working your upper body. Choose one exercise to work each of the six major muscle groups of your torso and arms (chest, shoulders, back, biceps, triceps, abs). For example, you might do bench presses, dumbbell side laterals, lat pull-downs (or chin-ups), biceps curls, triceps push-downs, and sit-ups. Your second workout of the week involves an indoor or outdoor cardio exercise of your choice to burn fat and shape your legs. Choose from exercises such as cycling, walking, jogging, or stair climbing.

IMPROVISE

The problem: Lack of facilities.

The solution: Adapt.

Let's assume you don't have access to gym facilities. You might be working away from home, out of town on business, visiting relatives, in the process of relocating, or just temporarily in the middle of nowhere. Bottom line? Your environment has changed, and you are lacking gym equipment. Maybe you've got a barbell or some dumbbells. Perhaps you have no equipment at all. So what does a guy do in the face of adversity? Improvise—adapt.

A basic barbell and some thoughtful improvisation are all you need to give any muscle a decent dose of iron. Let me give you an example of how to adapt to your circumstances and create a barbell-only shoulder-shocking routine. You have a choice of several barbell exercises for shoulders. But remember, if you're looking to build a solid set of cannonballs, your shoulder routine must target all three heads of the deltoid: front, side, and rear. Here's my suggestion for a barbell-only shoulder-shocking routine of four exercises to hit the deltoid from multiple angles. First up is *barbell front raise* to target the front deltoid. Take a shoulder-width overhand grip on the bar, loaded with a weight that allows you to perform eight repetitions. Upon completion, proceed immediately to exercise two, *barbell upright rows*, and bang out another eight reps to hit the lateral deltoid and trapezius. Next switch to a wide grip, bend forward at the waist, and perform a set of *bent-over barbell rows*. Squeeze out another eight reps, pulling the bar up toward your chest to target the rear delts. Finish with a set of *barbell shoulder presses* until you reach failure.

Performing these four shoulder exercises back to back, as a giant superset, is the way to go, especially if your supply of weights is limited. The sequence begins with the weakest exercise and proceeds through progressively stronger movements. Because each section of the deltoid gets roasted as you proceed through the exercise sequence, you probably won't need to change the weight on the barbell. You can of course perform this routine in a standard fashion of four separate exercises, but you will require a sufficient supply of weights to load the bar during the row and press exercises.

What if you don't even have a set of weights? Well, let me show you how to adapt the basic push-up to create a pectoral-pulverizing routine. The push-up is a great upper body exercise that targets the chest, shoulders, and triceps. The standard version of the floor push-up is performed with your hands placed directly beneath your shoulders. This standard position hits more fibers of the pectoral muscles than variations do. A narrow-base push-up with your hands placed less than shoulder-width apart activates the inner portion of the pectorals that helps define the separation down the center of your chest. A wide-base push-up with your hands positioned more than shoulder-width apart increases the stretch on the pectoral, which helps develop the outer portion of your chest. What's more, a narrow base maximizes triceps contribution, whereas a wide-base reduces involvement of the triceps. If you perform a decline push-up with your feet on a bench, you will target the upper pectorals. When you perform an incline push-up on your knees, you'll work the lower fibers of your chest. The incline push-up can also be performed with your feet on the floor and your hands positioned on a bench or chair. Note that your body position and muscular trajectory during the incline push-up resembles the *decline* bench press and during the decline push-up is similar to the *incline* bench press.

TRAVEL TIPS

To prevent those business trips (or vacations) from disrupting your workout program and diet, my top travel tip is go prepared. Maintaining dietary discipline during travel is not difficult if you use some convenient nutritional supplements. Before leaving home, pack a 24- to 48-hour supply of quality supplements. For the plane ride, pack a couple of ready-to-drink protein shakes and a handful of protein bars. Make sure to drink lots of water on the plane, which can help prevent jet lag. Pack as many sachets of meal-replacement powder as you can carry in your checked luggage. These are lifesavers when you arrive at your destination because the powder mixes easily with water in your hotel room.

If you're away for more than a couple of days, check the phone book for the nearest health food store so you can restock on supplements. This way you don't have to overload your luggage. During your hotel stay, try to find a grocery store for some easy-to-eat items such as cans or packets of water-packed tuna and a carton of nonfat milk. In most cities, you can hunt down at least one or two restaurants that cater to the health conscious.

As for exercise, most good hotels have an exercise room. Bring your lightweight workout gear. Even with the busiest of schedules, you should be able to fit in 30 minutes on the stationary bicycle. If the hotel health spa isn't to your liking, check the phone book to see if there's a good gym in town. If you're in a motel in the middle of nowhere, you'll have to make do with a brisk 30-minute walk or swim and maybe some push-ups and sit-ups. A little exercise is better than none at all.

The bottom line when traveling is that you can maintain an element of discipline in your diet and exercise routine with some thoughtful planning.

Now let's discuss degree of difficulty. During the standard push-up, with your hands and feet positioned on the ground, you lift approximately 66 percent (two-thirds) of your body weight. An incline push-up on your knees is easier, since you lift around 50 percent (one-half) of your body weight. A decline push-up with your feet on a bench is the hardest version, forcing you to lift approximately 75 percent (three-quarters) of your body weight. So performing a decline push-up followed immediately by a standard push-up and then an incline push-up is much like doing a triple drop set. Bottom line: Utilizing these push-up variations allows you to hit your chest from every angle and alter the relative resistance.

PLAN FOR LONGEVITY

The problem: getting older.

The solution: sculpting safely.

Like it or not, as your body ages it slowly deteriorates. So what happens? Your testosterone level decreases and your metabolism slows down at a rate of 10 percent per decade after age 30. The muscles and tendons become stiffer, less elastic, and more prone to injury. It also takes your body longer to recover after each workout. Hence, it makes good biological sense to adjust your training regimen as you get older. After all, you don't want to provoke pain in your shoulders, back, and knees or risk the possibility of a torn muscle or a rotator cuff injury. Here are my top 10 tips to aid longevity in the gym for men over 40.

1. Always warm up well.
2. Use higher reps (10 to 20 per set) with lighter weights.
3. Perform slow, steady movements.
4. Avoid extreme ranges of motion (overstretching).
5. Make use of machines (safer than free weights).
6. Shorten rest intervals to boost cardiorespiratory effort.
7. Use drop sets for added intensity, avoiding forced reps and negatives.
8. Allow ample recovery time between workouts.
9. Keep your rotator cuff strong.
10. Keep your core (abs and lower back) strong.

PUMP UP MOTIVATION

The problem: a poor attitude.

The solution: get motivated.

If you don't believe you can make progress, chances are you won't. You need a strong conviction in your ability. Believe that you're capable of more, and you'll achieve it. Lack of conviction will slowly infect all aspects of your exercise and nutrition program. It influences your intensity, dampens your discipline, and lets you neglect nutrition. Lack of motivation has a domino effect, knocking down all aspects of your progress.

Do everything in your power to control your attitude. Eliminate doubts or negative thoughts that might be holding you back, preventing you from reaching your full potential. Following are some of the ABCs of self-motivation.

Action Now that you've read this book, you have the knowledge you need to develop the ultimate body. Knowledge is indeed the key, but you have to put the key in the lock, open the door, and make it happen. It's easy to talk the talk, but you also must walk the walk. Turn your thoughts into action. Actions speak louder than words, and you must act to get the job done. Why dawdle? You have been wanting this for years. Do it.

Belief Believe to achieve. Everyone has potential—you've just got to make it happen. Snooze and lose. Strive and come alive. Use the bumper sticker that works for you. Believe in yourself and your capabilities. Nearly anything is possible if you want it badly enough.

Consistency Nothing happens overnight. It takes great willpower to stick with an exercise program and change your dietary habits, but you've got to stick with it. You have to be consistent, persistent, and patient. Great things come to those who wait. The change will happen; just give it a chance. To help yourself be consistent, make your workout schedule convenient. Select a time of day that works best for you; choose a gym that's conveniently located. The farther you have to travel to the gym, the less likely you'll make the journey. Don't give yourself any excuses.

Discipline   We're all creatures of habit. No matter how flexible you are, I bet there's some element of routine in your day-to-day living, a basic structure around which everything else revolves. We eat, drink, and sleep every day. Most of us have to work to earn a living, and we fit in some play time when possible. Without structure, there's chaos. Without rules, there's disorder. To build a better body, all you must do is make slight adjustments to your daily routine. Just add that little extra bit of discipline. Squeeze in a 30-minute workout; sprinkle some healthy spice into your diet. Come on, it's easy! If I can do it, anyone can. Take small steps at first. Just keep saying to yourself, "I can do this. I will do this. I have the discipline it takes."

Evolution   Your body evolves, and you have to change with it. You'll become stronger, fitter, and ready to rise to the next level to meet new challenges. It's all about progress. If you're not making progress, step back and take a critical look at what's holding you back. Isolate the problem and fix it. Don't get stuck in a rut. Keep moving up the ladder. Strive to climb farther up the hill; the view just gets better and better.

Faults   We all have our faults. No one is perfect. Whatever happens, don't let faults or mistakes hold you back. If you were not blessed with meaty arms, and they won't grow as fast as you'd like, don't throw in the towel. Rethink your arm workout; change your exercises. Maybe you're not using the right bait. Try to keep your exercise program and diet as simple as possible. Don't make something more complicated than it has to be. Some people suffer from information overload. They accumulate so much that they end up getting confused and can't see the forest for the trees. Simple exercise and diet regimens are often more effective than complicated ones. If you do make a mistake—miss a workout or binge on pizza—don't fret. What's done is done. Acknowledge your mistake and learn from it—then cast it aside and get back to your program.

Goals   Nothing is more motivating than witnessing progress. Scoring a goal is a great feeling, a reward for your efforts. But to reach a goal, you must set it in the first place. Without goals, you have no direction. To make your goal real, be diligent with documentation. When you keep a weekly record of measurements, such as strength, body weight, and body fat percentage, you can accurately chart your progress. Quick, objective measurements like these are better than subjective impressions, such as looking in the mirror, where visible changes tend to occur more slowly. If you want a regular income of motivation, set and record your short-term goals. Be realistic, take small steps at first, and enjoy monitoring your progress.

Finally, one last word. Enjoy. To do something regularly, you need to enjoy it. If you enjoy your exercise program, you won't need further motivation. Do everything in your power to make your workout experience enjoyable. Join a gym with a good atmosphere, train with a motivated workout buddy, or listen to your favorite tunes on a personal music player. Choose exercises that you actually like doing; if you enjoy the exercise, it will work for you. Enjoy your gym time. Sculpt your body. Stay healthy. Be happy. Start now. That's a doctor's order.

Appendix A

Training, Progress, and Nutrition Charts

Make copies of the following charts to plan and record your workouts, diet, and progress.

Training Log

Date	Muscle	Exercise	Set 1 (weight × reps)	Set 2 (weight × reps)	Set 3 (weight × reps)

Notes:

Workout time:

From N. Evans, 2011, *Men's Body Sculpting*, 2nd ed. (Champaign, IL: Human Kinetics).

Personal Diet Chart

Meal	Time	Food	Calories	Protein	Carbohydrate	Fat
1.						
2.						
3.						
4.						
5.						
6.						
		Totals (per day)				

From N. Evans, 2011, *Men's Body Sculpting*, 2nd ed. (Champaign, IL: Human Kinetics).

Progress Chart

Measurement	Time						
	Start	1 month	2 months	3 months	4 months	5 months	6 months
Body weight							
% body fat							
Size (inches/cm) Waist Chest Arms Thighs							
Cardio time							
Strength (6 reps) Bench press Squat Biceps curl							

Notes:

Appendix B

Food Nutrition Facts

Values are approximate. Check the nutrition facts label on individual brands. These foods are featured in the sample meal plans in chapters 7, 10, and 14. Protein foods are listed first, followed by sources of starchy carbohydrate and fibrous carbohydrate.

Food	Protein	Carbohydrate	Fat	Calories
Chicken breast (6 oz; 175 g)	35	0	6	200
Lean beef (6 oz; 175 g)	35	0	6	200
Turkey breast (6 oz; 175 g)	35	0	3	180
Tuna, water packed (6 oz; 175 g)	35	0	2	160
Egg white (1)	6	0	0	24
Nonfat milk (240 ml)	9	12	0	90
Rice (50 g)	3	39	0	170
Pasta (50 g)	6	40	1	200
Potato (1 medium)	2	35	0	150
Oats (40 g)	5	27	3	150
Carrots (80 g)	1	9	0	40
Broccoli (80 g)	1	4	0	20
Spinach (80 g)	2	3	0	20
Whole-wheat bread (1 slice)	4	18	2	110
Low-fat granola	4	36	4	200

Bibliography

EXERCISE AND MUSCLE HYPERTROPHY

Campos, G.E., Luecke, T.J., Wendeln, H.K., Toma, K., Hagerman, F.C., Murray, T.F., Ragg, K.E., Ratamess, N.A., Kraemer, W.J., and Staron, R.S. 2002. Muscular adaptations in response to three different resistance-training regimens: Specificity of repetition maximum training zones. *Eur J Appl Physiol* 88:50-60.

Chestnut, J.L., and Docherty, D. 1999. The effect of 4 and 10 repetition maximum weight-training protocols on neuromuscular adaptations in untrained men. *J Strength Cond Res* 13:353-359.

Gibala, M.J., Interisano, S.A., Tarnopolsky, M.A., Roy, B.D., MacDonald, J.R., Yarasheski, K.E., and MacDougall, J.D. 2000. Myofibrillar disruption following acute concentric and eccentric resistance exercise in strength-trained men. *Can J Physiol Pharmacol* 78:656-661.

Hass, C.J., Garzarella, L., de Hoyos, D., and Pollock, M.L. 2000. Single versus multiple sets in long-term recreational weightlifters. *Med Sci Sports Exerc* 32:235-242.

Kraemer, W.J., Marchitelli, L., Gordon, S.E., Harman, E., Dziados, J.E., Mello, R., Frykman, P., McCurry, D., and Fleck, S.J. 1990. Hormonal and growth factor response to heavy resistance exercise protocols. *J Appl Physiol* 69:1442-1450.

Kramer, J.B., Stone, M.H., O'Bryant, H.S., Conley, M.S., Johnson, R.L., Nieman, D.C., Honeycutt, D.R., and Hoke, T.P. 1997. Effects of single vs. multiple sets of weight training: Impact of volume, intensity, and variation. *J Strength Cond Res* 11:143-147.

MacDougall, J.D., Gibala, M.J., Tarnopolsky, M.A., MacDonald, J.R., Interisano, S.A., and Yarasheski, K.E. 1995. The time course for elevated muscle protein synthesis following heavy resistance exercise. *Can J Appl Physiol* 20:480-486.

McCall, G.E., Byrnes, W.C., Dickinson, A., Pattany, P.M., and Fleck, S.J. 1996. Muscle fiber hypertrophy, hyperplasia, and capillary density in college men after resistance training. *J Appl Physiol* 81:2004-2012.

Rhea, M.R., Alvar, B.A., Ball, S.D., and Burkett, L.N. 2002. Three sets of weight training superior to 1 set with equal intensity for eliciting strength. *J Strength Cond Res* 16:525-529.

Westcott, W.L., Winett, R.A., Anderson, E.S., Wojcik, J.R., Loud, R.L., Cleggett, E., and Glover, S. 2001. Effects of regular and slow speed resistance training on muscle strength. *J Sports Med Phys Fitness* 41:154-158.

Williams, A.G., Ismail, A.N., Sharma, A., and Jones, D.A. 2002. Effects of resistance exercise volume and nutritional supplementation on anabolic and catabolic hormones. *Eur J Appl Physiol* 86:315-321.

ANABOLIC STEROIDS

Bhasin, S., Storer, T.W., Berman, N., Callegari, C., Clevenger, B., Phillips, J., Bunnell, T.J., Tricker, R., Shirazi, A., and Casaburi, R. 1996. The effects of supraphysiological doses of testosterone on muscle size and strength in normal men. *N Eng J Med* 335:1-7.

Bhasin, S., Woodhouse, L., Casaburi, R., Singh, A.B., Bhasin, D., Berman, N., Chen, X., Yarasheski, K.E., Magliano, L., Dzekov, C., Dzekov, J., Bross, R., Phillips, J., Sinha-Hikim, I., Shen, R., and Storer, T.W. 2001. Testosterone dose-response relationships in healthy young men. *Am J Physiol Endocrinol Metab* 281:E1172-E1181.

Evans, N.A. 1997. Gym and tonic: A profile of 100 male steroid users. *Br J Sports Med* 31:54-58.

Evans, N.A. 1997. Local complications of self-administered anabolic steroid injections. *Br J Sports Med* 31:349-350.

Evans, N.A., Bowrey, D.J., and Newman, G.R. 1998. Ultrastructural analysis of ruptured tendon from anabolic steroid users. *Injury* 29:769-773.

Evans, N.A. 2004. Anabolic steroids: Answers to the bigger questions. *J Musculoskel Med* 21:166-178.

Evans, N.A. 2004. Current concepts in anabolic-androgenic steroids. *Am J Sports Med* 32:534-542.

Evans, N.A., and Parkinson, A. 2006. Anabolic androgenic steroids: A survey of 500 users. *Med Sci Sports Exerc* 38:644-651.

Sinha-Hikim, I., Artaza, J., Woodhouse, L., Gonzalez-Cadavid, N., Singh, A.B., Lee, M.I., Storer, T.W., Casaburi, R., Shen, R., and Bhasin, S. 2002. Testosterone-induced increase in muscle size in healthy young men is associated with muscle fiber hypertrophy. *Am J Physiol Endocrinol Metab* 283:E154-E164.

Sturmi, J.E., and Diorio, D.J. 1998. Anabolic agents. *Clin Sports Med* 17:261-282.

NUTRITION AND SUPPLEMENTS

Boozer, C.N., Daly, P.A., Homel, P., Solomon, J.L., Blanchard, D., Nasser, J.A., Strauss, R., and Meredith, T. 2002. Herbal ephedra/caffeine for weight loss: A 6-month randomized safety and efficacy trial. *Int J Obes Relat Metab Disord* 26:593-604.

Brief, A.A., Maurer, S.G., and Di Cesare, P.E. 2001. Use of glucosamine and chondroitin sulphate in the management of osteoarthritis. *J Am Acad Orthop Surg* 9:71-78.

Broeder, C.E. 2003. Oral andro-related prohormone supplementation: Do the potential risks outweigh the benefits? *Can J Appl Physiol* 28:102-116.

Burke, D.G., Candow, D.G., Chilibeck, P.D., MacNeil, L.G., Roy, B.D., Tarnopolsky, M.A., and Ziegenfuss, T. 2008. Effects of creatine supplementation and resistance exercise training on muscle insulin-like growth factor in young adults. *Int J Sport Nutr Exerc Metab* 18:389-398.

Burke, D.G., Chilibeck, P.D., Davidson, K.S., Candow, D.G., Farthing, J., and Smith-Palmer, T. 2001. The effect of whey protein supplementation with and without creatine monohydrate combined with resistance training on lean tissue mass and muscle strength. *Int J Sport Nutr Exerc Metab* 11:349-364.

Catlin, D.H., Leder, B.Z., Ahrens, B., Starcevic, B., Hatton, C.K., Green, G.A., and Finkelstein, J.S. 2000. Trace contamination of over-the-counter androstenedione and positive urine test results for a nandrolone metabolite. *JAMA* 284:2618-2621.

Delbeke, F.T., Van Eenoo, P., Van Thuyne, W., and Desmet, N. 2003. Prohormones and sport. *J Steroid Biochem Mol Biol* 83:245-251.

King, D.S., Sharp, R.L., Vukovich, M.D., Brown, G.A., Reifenrath, T.A., Uhl, N.L., and Parsons, K.A. 1999. Effect of oral androstenedione on serum testosterone and adaptations to resistance training in young men. *JAMA* 281:2020-2028.

Kreider, R.B., Melton, C., Rasmussen, C.J., Greenwood, M., Lancaster, S., Cantler, E.C., Milnor, P., and Almada, A.L. 2003. Long-term creatine supplementation does not significantly affect clinical markers of health in athletes. *Mol Cell Biochem* 244:95-104.

Lawrence, M.E., and Kirby, D.F. 2002. Nutrition and sports supplements: Fact or fiction. *J Clin Gastroenterol* 35:299-306.

Leder, B.Z., Longcope, C., Catlin, D.H., Ahrens, B., Schoenfeld, D.A., and Finkelstein, J.S. 2000. Oral androstenedione administration and serum testosterone concentrations in young men. *JAMA* 283:779-782.

Nissen, S.L., and Sharp, R.L. 2003. Effect of dietary supplements on lean mass and strength gains with resistance exercise: A meta-analysis. *J Appl Physiol* 94:651-659.

Rawson, E.S., and Volek, J.S. 2003. Effects of creatine supplementation and resistance training on muscle strength and weightlifting performance. *J Strength Cond Res* 17:822-831.

Reginster, J.Y., Deroisy, R., Rovati, L.C., Lee, R.L., Lejeune, E., Bruyere, O., Giacovelli, G., Henrotin, Y., Dacre, J.E., and Gossett, C. 2001. Long-term effects of glucosamine sulphate on osteoarthritis progression: A randomized placebo-controlled trial. *Lancet* 357:251-256.

Roy, B.D., Fowles, J.R., Hill, R., and Tarnopolsky, M.A. 2000. Macronutrient intake and whole body protein metabolism following resistance exercise. *Med Sci Sports Exerc* 32:1412-1418.

Rozenek, R., Ward, P., Long, S., and Garhammer, J. 2002. Effects of high-calorie supplementation on body composition and muscular strength following resistance training. *J Sports Med Phys Fitness* 42:340-347.

Schedel, J.M., Tanaka, H., Kiyonaga, A., Shindo, M., and Schutz, Y. 2000. Acute creatine loading enhances human growth hormone secretion. *J Sports Med Phys Fitness* 40:336-342.

Shekelle, P.G., Hardy, M.L., Morton, S.C., Maglione, M., Mojica, W.A., Suttorp, M.J., Rhodes, S.L., Jungvig, L., and Gagne, J. 2003. Efficacy and safety of ephedra and ephedrine for weight loss and athletic performance. *JAMA* 289:1537-1545.

Silver, M.D. 2001. Use of ergogenic aids by athletes. *J Am Acad Orthop Surg* 9:61-70.

Tarnopolsky, M.A., Atkinson, S.A., MacDougall, J.D., Chesley, A., Phillips, S., and Schwarcz, H.P. 1992. Evaluation of protein requirements for trained strength athletes. *J Appl Physiol* 73:1986-1995.

Tarnopolsky, M.A., Parise, G., Yardley, N.J., Ballantyne, C.S., Olatinji, S., and Phillips, S.M. 2001. Creatine-dextrose and protein-dextrose induce similar strength gains during training. *Med Sci Sports Exerc* 33:2044-2052.

Terjung, R.L., Clarkson, P., Eichner, E.R., Greenhaff, P.L., Hespel, P.J., Israel, R.G., Kraemer, W.J., Meyer, R.A., Spriet, L.L., Tarnopolsky, M.A., Wagenmakers, A.J., and Williams, M.H. 2000. American College of Sports Medicine roundtable. The physiological and health effects of oral creatine supplementation. *Med Sci Sports Exerc* 32:706-717.

Vierck, J.L., Icenoggle, D.L., Bucci, L., and Dodson, M.V. 2003. The effects of ergogenic compounds on myogenic satellite cells. *Med Sci Sports Exerc* 35:769-776.

Volek, J.S., Duncan, N.D., Mazzetti, S.A., Staron, R.S., Putukian, M., Gomez, A.L., Pearson, D.R., Fink, W.J., and Kraemer, W.J. 1999. Performance and muscle fiber adaptations to creatine supplementation and heavy resistance training. *Med Sci Sports Exerc* 31:1147-1156.

Volek, J.S., and Rawson, E.S. 2004. Scientific basis and practical aspects of creatine supplementation for athletes. *Nutrition* 20:609-614.

Wallace, M.B., Lim, J., Cutler, A., and Bucci, L. 1999. Effects of dehydroepiandrosterone vs. androstenedione supplementation in men. *Med Sci Sports Exerc* 31:1788-1792.

Ziegenfuss, T.N., Berardi, J.M., and Lowery, L.M. 2002. Effects of prohormone supplementation in humans: A review. *Can J Appl Physiol* 27:628-646.

Index

Note: Page references followed by an italicized *f* or *t* indicate information contained in figures and tables, respectively.

A

abdominal muscles
  anatomy 35*ft*-36
  body fat blitz program 113-114, 119-120
  exercises for 50*t*, 51-52
  hybrid hard body program 162-163, 185-186
  mass generator program 72, 80
  "six-pack" 88-89
adaptation, muscle 4-5
addiction, steroid 138
adenosine triphosphate (ATP) 4
age, and training 225-226
alcohol 96-97
amino acids 54
anabolic state
  about 53
  anabolic window 56
  and body type 60
  caloric balance 54-55
  carbohydrates and 54
  cardio workouts 57
  growth hormone 59
  insulin 59-60
  proteins and 54
  rest and recovery 55-56
  supplements 56-57
  testosterone boosting 57-58
  water and 55
anaerobic energy sources 4-5
androstenedione 148
arm muscles. *See also specific arm muscles*
  anatomy 31*f*-32*ft*
  body fat blitz program 111-112
  exercises for 50*t*, 52
Aspirin 146-147
asymmetry 196

B

B, vitamin 20, 21
back muscles
  anatomy 30*t*
  body fat blitz program 109-110
  exercises for 50*t*, 51
  hybrid hard body program 164-166
  mass generator program 77-78
back safety 209-210

biceps
  anatomy 31*f*
  biceps blast 128-129
  exercises for 50*t*
  hybrid hard body program 167-168
  mass generator program 79
  sculpting 193
biological value (BV) 17
body fat blitz program
  about 99-101
  exercises 105-120
  nutrition plan 101-103, 102*t*
  progress measurement 103
  results 103
  summary 104
body mass index (BMI) 38-39, 38*t*, 40*t*, 96
body types 37-39, 38*t*, 60, 98
brachialis 31*f*
brachioradialis 31*f*

C

C, vitamin 20, 21
caffeine 94, 146-147
calcium 20-21
calf muscles
  anatomy 34
  body fat blitz program 118
  exercises for 50*t*
  hybrid hard body program 176-177
  mass generator program 76
caloric balance 14, 84-87, 92
calories 14
carbohydrate 13, 16*t*, 18-19, 18*t*, 54, 92
cardiorespiratory workouts
  avoiding 57
  body fat blitz program 113, 119
  and fat loss 92
  high-speed cardio 87, 87*t*
  hybrid hard body program 171, 187
  using for weight loss 84
catabolism 57
chest muscles
  anatomy 28*ft*
  body fat blitz program 105-106
  chest chiseling 129
  exercises 49-50, 50*t*
  hybrid hard body program 157-159
  mass generator program 67-68

cholesterol 20
cleanliness and hygiene 221-222
clenbuterol 136
coffees, flavored 96-97
colds 223
compound exercise 47
concentric muscle contraction 6-7
creatine 23, 146

D

data recording 40
dehydro epiandrosterone (DHEA) 148
deltoids
    anatomy 29*f*
    deltoid demolition 128
    hybrid hard body program 181-183
    sculpting 191-193
Dianabol 136
diet and nutrition
    caloric balance 14
    caloric balance and anabolic state 54-55
    components of 13-21, 17*t*, 18*t*, 20*t*
    dietary discipline 218-220
    for extra leanness 199-200, 199*t*
    for fat loss 97
    food nutrition facts 233
    hybrid hard body program 153, 154*t*
    mass generator program 62-64, 63*t*
    meal planning and preparation 21-25, 22*t*, 88
    nutrients 16-21, 17*t*, 18*t*, 20*t*
    personal diet chart 231
    for "six-pack" abdominals 88-89
    spices 24
    timing 14-16
diuretics 136
drop sets 125

E

E, vitamin 20, 21
eccentric muscle contraction 6-7
echinacea 149
ectomorph body type 37, 38, 40*t*, 60, 98
elbow safety 210
endomorph body type 37, 38, 40*t*, 60, 98
endurance *vs.* strength 4, 7
ephedrine 136, 146-147
erector spinae 30
essential fatty acids 20
exercises
    abdomen 35*t*, 50*t*
    arms 32*t*, 50*t*
    back 30*t*, 50*t*
    biceps 50*t*
    calves 50*t*
    chest 28*t*, 50*t*
    exercise finder vi-vii
    forearms 50*t*
    hamstrings 50*t*
    legs 35*t*
    quadriceps 50*t*
    shoulders 29*t*, 50*t*
    triceps 50*t*

F

fat, dietary 13, 19-20, 20*t*
fat burner supplements 146-148, 147*t*
fat loss
    alcohol 96-97
    and body types 98
    diet considerations 97
    exercise window for 93
    extra leanness 199-200, 199*t*
    hormone balance 93
    rule of three Cs 92-93
    sleep and 95-96
    speed workouts 94-95
    spot reducing 97
    supplements 94
    thermogenic drugs and supplements 136, 146-147
    waist reduction 95
fat tissue 11, 83
fiber, dietary 19
first aid 204
flexibility 11
focused contraction training (FCT) 45-46
food nutrition facts 233
forearm muscles
    anatomy 32*f*
    exercises for 50*t*
    hybrid hard body program 169-170
    sculpting 195
free weights 51
fructose 18-19
fruits 18-19
fuel, muscle
    about 4, 10, 13
    components of diet 13-22, 17*t*, 18*t*, 20*t*, 22*t*

G

Garcinia cambogia 94
ghrelin 96
ginseng 149
glucosamine 148
glucose 18
glutamine 23, 130
gluteus maximus 34, 195
glycemic index 18

glycogen 4
green tea 94
growth hormone (GH) 56, 59, 93, 136-137
guarana 147
gynecomastia 138

H

hamstrings
    anatomy 33*f*, 34
    body fat blitz program 117
    exercises for 50*t*
    hybrid hard body program 174-175
    mass generator program 75
heart rate 85
herbs, as supplements 149
high-speed cardio 87, 87*t*
hip safety 212
hoodia 89, 94, 147*t*
hormone balance 93
human chorionic gonadotropin (HCG) 136
hybrid hard body program
    about 151
    exercises 157-187
    nutrition plan 153, 154*t*
    progress measurements 155
    results 155
    summary 156
    workout plan 151-153
hydration 13, 21, 55
hypertrophic adaptation 4, 7-8

I

injuries
    about 201
    causes 201-202
    elbow safety 210
    first aid 204
    hip safety 212
    joint protection 206-207
    knee safety 212-213
    muscle care 205-206
    neck safety 207
    prevention 202-203
    shoulder safety 208-210, 209*t*
    spine safety 210-211
    stretching 206
    tendon care 204-205
insulin 59-60, 136
intensity of workout
    about 123, 221
    hyperintensity training 127-129
    rules 129-131
    steps to raise 123-127
interval training 87, 87*t*

isolation exercise 47
isometric muscle contraction 6-7, 126

J

joint protection 206-207

K

knee safety 212-213

L

laboratory tests 140, 141*t*
lactic acid 4-5
latissimus dorsi 30
leg muscles. *See also specific leg muscles*
    anatomy 33*f*-34*f*, 35*t*
    exercises for 50*t*, 52
leptin 96

M

machines, weight 51
macronutrients 13
ma-huang 147
mass generator program
    about 61
    caloric intake 64*t*
    exercises 67-80
    frequency 62
    nutrition plan 62-64, 63*t*
    progress measurement 64
    results 65
    summary 66
    workout plan 62
meal-replacement products 145
mesomorph body type 37, 38, 40*t*, 60, 98
metabolic adaptation 4, 7
Methandrostenolone 136
micronutrients 20
minerals and vitamins 20-21
motivation 226-227
muscle anatomy
    abdominals 35*f*-36
    arms 31*f*-32*f*
    back 30
    chest 28*f*
    full body diagram 27*f*
    legs 33*f*-34*f*
    proportion 48-49
    shoulders 29*f*
    size and exercise number 47-49
muscle care 205-206
muscle contraction 6-7
muscle growth 4-5, 197-198
muscle memory 216
muscle soreness 130

N

nandrolone decanoate 136
neck safety 207
needle injection issues 139-140
negative repetitions 126-127
neural adaptation 4, 7
Nolvadex 136
norandrostenedione 148

O

omega-3 and -6 20
overload 5
oxygen 4

P

pectoralis major 28f, 203
personal diet chart 231
phosphocreatine 4
polypharmacy 135-136
prefatiguing 124-125
PRICED first aid 204
programs of training, planning
    adapting 41
    body types 37-39
    data recording 40
    exercise number 47-49
    exercise order 47
    exercise selection 49-52, 50t
    exercise types 47
    selecting 39-40, 40t
    upgrading and modifying 41-42
progress chart 232
prohormones 148
protein 13, 17-18, 17t, 18t, 54
protein supplement 145
pump 197-198
push-ups 225

Q

quadriceps
    anatomy 33f
    body fat blitz program 115-116
    exercises for 50t
    hybrid hard body program 171-173
    mass generator program 73-74
    sculpting 193-194

R

range of motion 46
recovery 11-12
repair, muscle 4
repetition, precision 6-8, 7t
repetition tempo 125-126

rotator cuff
    anatomy 29f
    hybrid hard body program 178-180
    safety issues 209t
rowing 86

S

saturated fat 20
sculpting, advanced. *See also* training, weight
    about 191
    asymmetry 196
    biceps 193
    deltoids 191-193
    extra leanness 199-200, 199t
    forearms 194-195
    gluteus maximus 195
    plateaus 197
    pump 197-198
    quadriceps 195-196
    triceps 193-194
    vascularity 198
    v-shape taper 196-197
serratus anterior 28f
sets, lifting 8-10
shin splints 211
shoulder muscles
    anatomy 29ft
    body fat blitz program 107-108
    exercises for 50t, 51
    mass generator program 69-70
    rotator cuff program 178-180
    rotator cuff safety 209t
shoulder safety 208-210, 209t
skin changes 138
sleep 56, 95-96, 220-221
soda 19
somatotropin 136-137
speed workouts 94-95
spine safety 210-211
sport nutrition 143
spot reducing 97
spotters 9
St. John's wort 149
steroids
    about 133
    action 133-134
    doses and regimens 134-135, 135t
    injection issues 139-140
    lab tests 140, 141t
    polypharmacy and 135-136
    reasons to avoid 141-142
    side effects and health risks 136-138, 137t
stimulus 4, 7

stretching 130, 206
sucrose 18
supersets 95, 125
supplements, nutritional
about 56-57
creatine 146
fat burners 146-148, 147*t*
and fat loss 94
glucosamine 148
herbs 149
meal-replacement products 145
multivitamins and minerals 149
prohormones 148
protein 145
reasons for using 143-144
selecting 150
summary of 144*t*
Sustanon 250 136
Synthol 136

T

tamoxifen 136
tendon care 204-205
tendon injury 138
testicle shrinkage 137
testosterone
boosting 56, 57-58
and fat loss 93
in steroids 133-134
thermogenic drugs and supplements 136, 146-147
thigh muscles 33*f*
thyroid hormone 136
training, weight. *See also* sculpting, advanced
age and 225-226
for body types 37-39
dietary discipline 218-220
downtime 222-223
focus and distractions 221
hyperintensity training 127-129
intensification 123-127, 129-131
periodization 217-218, 217*t*
plateaus 197
precision repetition 6-8, 7*t*
program prescription 37-42, 38*t*, 40*t*
progress chart 232
proportional sculpting 216-217
recovery 11-12
rest intervals 10, 124
rules 5-12, 7*t*
selecting program of 39-40, 40*t*

speed workouts 94-95
supersets 95
training log 230
and travel 225
variety in 215-216
workout time 10-11, 15, 23, 93
work sets 8-9
training log 230
training volume 8
trans fat 20
trapezius 30, 184
travel, and training 225
triceps
anatomy 31*f*
exercises for 50*t*
hybrid hard body program 160-161
mass generator program 71
sculpting 194-195
Type II muscle fibers 4
Type I muscle fibers 4

V

vascularity 198
vegetables 19
vitamins and minerals 20-21, 149
v-shape taper 196-197

W

waist reduction 95
water 13, 21, 55
weather effects 218
weight loss
alcohol 96-97
and body types 98
caloric balance for 84-87
diet considerations 97
exercise window for 93
high-speed cardio 87, 87*t*
hormone balance 93
rule of three Cs 92-93
"six-pack" abdominals 88-89
sleep and 95-96
speed workouts 94-95
spot reducing 97
supplements 94
waist reduction 95
whey protein 145
willow bark 147
workout time 10-11
wrist pain 195

About the Author

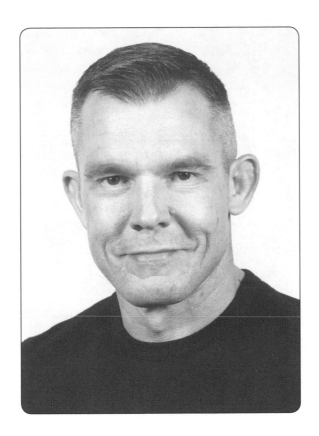

Nick Evans, BSc, MD, FRCS *(Orth)*, is an orthopedic surgeon specializing in sport injury. He studied medicine at the University of London, England, and trained in orthopedic surgery at the University Hospital of Wales. Evans gained additional skills in arthroscopic surgery at the Southern California Center for Sports Medicine and the University of California at Los Angeles.

Evans is a highly regarded authority on strength training, nutrition, and weight training injuries. He has fostered research in sport injury and performance enhancement and has written for many scientific publications. Evans is the author of *Bodybuilding Anatomy* and was a regular columnist for *MuscleMag International* and *Oxygen Women's Fitness* magazines. He is also featured in several weight training instructional DVDs.

Nick Evans practices and resides in North Yorkshire, England.

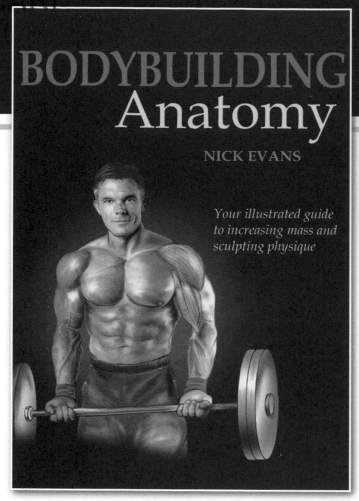